GIVING IT TO YOU
STRAIGHT

EVERYTHING YOU EVER WANTED
TO KNOW ABOUT **ORTHODONTICS** BUT
WERE AFRAID TO ASK

GIVING IT TO YOU
STRAIGHT

SETH NEWMAN, DDS & EFSTATHIOS GIANNOUTSOS, DDS

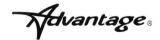

Published by Advantage, Charleston, South Carolina.
Member of Advantage Media Group.

ADVANTAGE is a registered trademark, and the Advantage colophon is a trademark of Advantage Media Group, Inc.

Printed in the United States of America.

10 9 8 7 6 5 4 3 2 1

ISBN: 978-1-59932-901-7
LCCN: 2018962238

Cover design by Melanie Cloth.
Layout design by Megan Elger.

This publication is designed to provide accurate and authoritative information in regard to the subject matter covered. It is sold with the understanding that the publisher is not engaged in rendering legal, accounting, or other professional services. If legal advice or other expert assistance is required, the services of a competent professional person should be sought.

Advantage Media Group is proud to be a part of the Tree Neutral® program. Tree Neutral offsets the number of trees consumed in the production and printing of this book by taking proactive steps such as planting trees in direct proportion to the number of trees used to print books. To learn more about Tree Neutral, please visit **www.treeneutral.com**.

Advantage Media Group is a publisher of business, self-improvement, and professional development books and online learning. We help entrepreneurs, business leaders, and professionals share their Stories, Passion, and Knowledge to help others Learn & Grow. Do you have a manuscript or book idea that you would like us to consider for publishing? Please visit **advantagefamily.com** or call **1.866.775.1696**.

To moms and dads everywhere, and to our team,
without whom we could not do this.

TABLE OF CONTENTS

ACKNOWLEDGMENTS

This book wouldn't have been possible without the love and support of our parents, our wives, and our six wonderful children (we have three each), as well as the doctors who dedicated their time teaching us at the NYU College of Dentistry. Furthermore, we couldn't have created the wonderful smiles we see from our patients every day without the support of our entire staff. Every one of you make it possible and worthwhile for us to do what we do.

Thank You!

—Drs. Giannoutsos & Newman

FOREWORD

In an age of questionable, disseminated health information presented to the public and to the medical and dental professions at large via the Internet, it is refreshing to see an invaluable resource for adult patients, parents of young patients, teenage patients, dentists, and physicians.

Giving It to You Straight: Everything You Ever Wanted to know about Orthodontics but Were Afraid to Ask by Drs. Efstathios Giannoutsos and Seth Newman covers an extraordinary breadth of the way modern orthodontics should be practiced. Each chapter has been well researched and represents the most current evidence-based information as well as time honored "best practices" anecdotal experience.

The authors themselves are well qualified to write such an important book that will be easily read and understood by the public. Drs. Giannoutsos and Newman were outstanding residents in the orthodontic program at The New York University College of Dentistry and demonstrated a high level of both technical and academic skills as well as strong ethical and moral obligations to the patients under their care. Teaming up after graduation, they enjoy a well-deserved reputation for having a premier orthodontic practice.

This book can be read in several ways. Firstly, it can be read from cover to cover (recommended) or, alternatively, used as a reference resource for the reader to select chapters of interest. Patients already under treatment can find information that will detail what lies ahead for them during and after their orthodontic treatment. For example, Chapter 8: Retention for Life will describe the reasons why retention of an orthodontic outcome requires continued vigilance by the orthodontist and the different types of holding devices (retainers) currently used in orthodontic practice.

The authors refrain from avoiding subjects that are rarely (but should be) covered prior to orthodontic treatment. For example, the types and degree of discomfort that patients may experience during orthodontic treatment, cost of orthodontic treatment, the qualifications of clinicians delivering an orthodontic service, and a rationale and compassionate protocol for making very young patients and their parents comfortable during the early visits to an orthodontic practice.

Giving It to You Straight: Everything You Ever Wanted to know about Orthodontics but Were Afraid to Ask will help debunk myths about orthodontic treatment which may persuade some patients to undergo orthodontic treatment and practical "in place" protocols used by the authors to demonstrate how an orthodontic practice and patients and parents should be managed. The reader will come away with a valuable, educational experience without perceiving the authors as self-promoting.

After carefully reviewing this book, I was very pleased to write this foreword as I consider this book to be a truthful, valid, educational, and practical tool for the public and the dental profession.

Elliott M. Moskowitz, DDS, MSd
Clinical Professor, Department of Orthodontics
NYU College of Dentistry
Diplomate of the American Board of Orthodontics

MEET THE DOCTORS

It's our hope that this book will give you a deeper understanding of what to expect as a patient or as the parent of a patient going through orthodontics. Even though we see most of our patients about every six weeks during their treatment, the success of each case depends just as much on what they do for themselves when they're not in our office as what we do for them when they are.

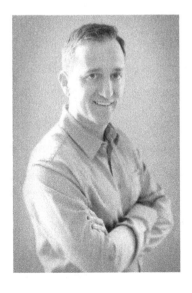

SETH NEWMAN, DDS

I grew up in Staten Island, New York, the son of a school teacher. My two uncles were general dentists and partners in a practice in Brooklyn and Manhattan. Growing up, I would spend a lot of time with my uncles in their offices. I could see that they really loved what they did. I think in some ways, being exposed to their partnership at an early age also taught me the value that a good partner could bring. One of my uncles even had a boat, which was a huge thing for a seven-year-old. When people asked me what I wanted to be when I grew up, I always said, "A dentist." When they asked why, I explained that it was "because I want to have a boat."

I started with premed at Binghamton and made my way into Stony Brook Dental School. In my first year, I tried to take in all the different areas of dentistry and kept an open mind. It wasn't until the second year, when we were exposed to the specializations, that I discovered orthodontics. The orthodontists generally seemed to like what they did, and I was intrigued by their focus on the art and science of straight, beautiful teeth.

Following dental school, I did a year of general residency at Mount Sinai, which was an invaluable confidence builder. While I was still at Mount Sinai, I was accepted to NYU for orthodontics, which was great, until two weeks later when I got my first tuition bill. Even in the early 2000s, it was already $53,000 for the year and I had no idea where I was going to get the money.

Then, one morning over coffee, I asked one of my mentors at Mount Sinai if he knew where I could get a job working as an associate for another doctor. He suggested I start a practice. Before I knew it, I was a dentist on the upper east side of Manhattan.

Even though it was a prestigious address, I truly was working a one-man show. I had to answer my own office phone and spent my nights filling out insurance claims and signing up for every insurance plan I could find.

The biggest challenge, however, was finding clients. Things were slow until one day I decided to try out Craigslist. I decided to list my services under the "free" section, where people posted things like "curb alerts" and free movie screenings, offering a "free dental exam and cleaning." Within an hour, I'd have forty appointments scheduled and I'd have to take the ad down as I couldn't handle all the calls.

Of those forty people, maybe a third of them would show up. I'd do the free cleaning and exam, and out of those, only a third would agree to do any of the work that I recommended. This went on weekend after weekend until I was able to build a practice. The first year I brought in about $30,000, but by the second year I'd built it to $104,000 and I was able to pay my NYU tuition without taking out any loans.

That second year at NYU was a game changer for me, not just because I gained the confidence to run and grow a practice, but because it was the year I met Efstathios "Steve" Giannoutsos. He was my little brother in NYU's big brother/little brother program and we hit it off from the start.

I decided to open a practice in Roslyn, New York, on a signature loan right after I graduated. Today, I realize how fortunate I was to have that option—it was pre-2008 recession and a signature loan basically mean that, as a doctor, all the bank needed was my name on the dotted line and I got all the funds I needed to open an office.

While I was plugging away in Roslyn and working other jobs on the side to pay the bills, Steve and I stayed in touch. About two years after I started my office in Roslyn, Steve called me up and got right to the point. "You want to buy a practice together?" he asked.

It turned out that an orthodontist cousin of his had a practice in Jackson Heights and he'd recently decided to leave the orthodontics practice. He wanted to sell his office and Steve came to mind as a potential buyer.

"Sure," I said and with that, we started our first practice together—Jackson Heights Orthodontics. We each gave up our side jobs and started working two days a week in the Jackson Heights location and the other days in our individual offices, and it just grew from there.

As we write this book, I'm forty years old and truly love working with all of our wonderful patients, and I look forward to coming in to work every day. The only thing is, I still don't have a boat.

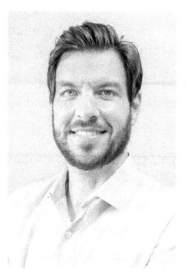

EFSTATHIOS GIANNOUTSOS, DDS

My entire family is from Greece. This is a place where dentistry has historically been, and continues to be, a major luxury. In the past, people couldn't have regular dental work due to geographic and social constraints. In such a historically agrarian society, they did not tend to themselves or their oral needs until their family's general welfare was taken care of and the land was tended to, or unless there was an emergency.

A memory that has stayed with me since my early childhood is that members of my family in Greece never smiled in pictures because so many of them had unsightly black, rotten, or missing teeth. There just was not enough money or enough time. Their lives were filled with farming; minding the tobacco fields; milking the sheep, goats and cows; and making cheese. Visiting the dentist was one of the last things on their minds.

I decided that I wanted to go into dentistry at the age of twelve, shortly after I got my braces. Money was tight, and my family didn't have the blessings we do today, so after a consultation with a private orthodontist, we discovered that we simply couldn't afford the treatment in a private practice and opted to go to the dental school at New York University (NYU).

After my treatment was completed at NYU, I kept in contact with some of the "resident" doctors who had treated me, and years later, after going to St. John's University, I found myself once again at NYU—this time as a dental student focused on graduating and going into orthodontics.

It was during one of the many times I was brown nosing in the orthodontic clinic that I met Seth Newman. We became great friends and worked so well together that we decided that we wanted to work together eventually.

He told me that he'd read about a practice for sale in Connecticut in the American Journal of Orthodontics and Dentofacial Orthopedics, and not only was it located only ten minutes from where we wanted to live, but it turned out that the seller was also my wife's former orthodontist. I called Dr. Norkin that evening while the bonfire on the Cape Cod beach was still smoldering and arranged to meet up. Early on what should have been the final day of the family vacation, I drove to Connecticut to meet with him and struck a deal. This was the only reason my lovely wife was willing to accept my bailing out on our time together. Thankfully, her parents had joined us in Cape Cod and were gracious enough to drive her and my daughters back to New York.

The practice in Connecticut picked up quickly, so I let the gentleman I had partnered with in Astoria take over most of the patients from our Astoria practice and absorb them into his busy Jackson Heights, Queens location. But then, a year later, I got a call from him telling me that he needed to sell for relocation purposes. He was leaving for service in the Marines, he said, and even though he was doing extraordinarily well, he wanted out. This was quite possibly the best bit of luck I had been graced with—and the seed for my success and partnership with Dr. Newman.

It was my opportunity to return a favor. I called Seth up and said, "Listen, you helped me find this Connecticut practice and now I have an opportunity for both of us—a practice that we can work in together."

He didn't hesitate. "I'm in; let's do it," he said. Typical Dr. Newman!

We bought the practice in Jackson Heights and that was that—the little ember that sparked the fire.

It was never my plan to run a practice, or even co-run one. I'd intended to continue working through reconstructive plastic surgery and spending most of my time focused on that, keeping my foot in the academic circles and bringing home a comfortable paycheck. But then the financial crisis of 2008 happened; we lost funding, and a lot of the opportunities that had been available before were now gone. But in tandem with Seth, we were able to flip those circumstances on their heads and use them to our advantage, and now I couldn't be happier with the direction we're going.

Seth and I have a profound mutual respect for each other's inherent skill sets, which are very complementary of each other. There are a few core areas where we overlap, but they're all overlaps in the right places: our work ethic, honesty to each other, and commitment to quality, for example. I know that sounds cliché, but these are real for us and in these places, we're almost the same person. These are our foundations, and from them we allow each other to stretch out and pursue our gifts, comfortable in the fact that we share common ground and can learn from each other's perspective.

CHAPTER 1

We Get You Straight and Dentists Keep You Healthy

By Seth Newman, DDS

Dr. Giannoutsos and I are truly appreciative of the dentists in our community. We couldn't be successful at orthodontics without them. They are our partners in treating each of our patients, providing valuable insight into the direction that our orthodontics should go, and taking responsibility for the health and well-being of our patients as we work to move their teeth. The open dialog we keep with dentists is what makes us truly successful in our profession.

It's not uncommon for us to come in for the day and have multiple emails, texts, and phone calls from dentists, each of them sending in a quick update on a patient that we're working on together or looking to have a discussion on the ongoing needs of our many mutual patients and their respective treatment needs.

One morning, I remember opening an email from Dr. Sami, a dentist in Queens, about a twelve-year-old patient he and I had been working with.

"Sara came in yesterday with decay at her gingival margins [her gum line]," it read. "I bonded it and did a full exam, and didn't see any other issues, but I also put her on a high fluoride toothpaste just to be safe. Her hygiene needs work, so just a head's up, and let's both watch her carefully!"

This is the kind of communication we love. I was concerned for Sara, of course—we'd have to talk more about the importance of thoroughly brushing around her braces when I saw her again—but it's that partnership with the dentist that makes it so much easier to keep up with our patients' health and keep them moving along with their treatment.

WHAT'S THE DIFFERENCE BETWEEN AN ORTHODONTIST AND A DENTIST?

Oftentimes there is a misconception about what an orthodontist does versus the role of a dentist. One doesn't take the place of the other—we work together to ensure the overall health and function of a person's mouth. For instance, patients often believe that orthodontists are cleaning their teeth and checking for cavities. While we'll certainly notice any obvious cavities, we don't have the focused imaging capabilities that dentists have for effectively diagnosing and treating cavities. Instead, our focus is on moving teeth, and we rely on our dental partners to keep our patients' teeth healthy.

Brian is a great example of this common misunderstanding. A nice guy in his mid-forties, Brian had been a particularly challenging case. He needed about eighteen months of clear braces to resolve severe crowding and an overbite. In the end, however, we had amazing results.

The day the braces came off, Brian smiled at me and said, "Doc, I can't thank you enough. My teeth look amazing and they've never been cleaner!"

I was puzzled.

"They do look great, but what do you mean by 'They've never been cleaner'?" I asked.

"Well, I know I'm supposed to go to the dentist twice a year and, I usually only go once—but you guys have been cleaning my teeth every six weeks, and they've never felt better," he said.

I gently explained to him the difference between orthodontists and dentists, and that we hadn't been cleaning his teeth for the past eighteen months. Then we gave Brian's dentist a call and set up an appointment for him later that week. No harm done, but it's surprising how common this misunderstanding can be.

Some other differences between dentists and orthodontists include:

- **Your first dental visit vs. your first orthodontic visit.**

You may not remember the first time you saw a dentist. Some patients see their dentist as early as six months old, or at the age of two. From that point on, they see their dentist every six months for regular cleanings and to make sure everything is coming in correctly. This early start with dentists has two big benefits:

1. *Patients are much more comfortable about seeing a dentist—and later, an orthodontist—because they're used to coming in for regular cleanings.*

When people see their dentist regularly, they generally don't run into big dental problems. Tooth decay and gum disease (both chronic conditions that usually take a long time to develop) are either prevented entirely or caught early, limiting any issues they may cause. And if they do develop a dental issue, such as a cavity, the condition will be caught early before it becomes a large problem.

2. *Dentists who see their patients regularly have the benefit of monitoring the growth and development of their patients' mouths and jaws. Over time, they're able to note what is normal dental development and what issues require further examination.*

Being able to monitor a patient's baby-tooth loss and adult-tooth development gives the dentist a much clearer idea of that patient's growth pattern, since there's no exact age when children lose their first baby teeth—just a range. If a child loses his or her teeth a little later than average, for instance, that time frame gives the dentist a better idea of when to expect the others to fall out, as growth patterns tend to remain consistent.

Then, once the patient is far enough along in dental development to see an orthodontist, the dentist can give the orthodontist a much better synopsis of the situation.

Patients are typically old enough to see an orthodontist at around seven or eight years old, most commonly at the recommendation of their dentist. However, we see plenty of astute parents who bring their children in because something just doesn't look right to them, or because someone else in the family has gone through orthodontics.

It could be because the parents noticed a crossbite or crowding of the teeth that might benefit from early treatment. Even if they don't see any immediate concerns developing in the mouth, it's recommended that children see an orthodontist around age seven or eight just to have a screening image done and to ensure that there are no issues developing.

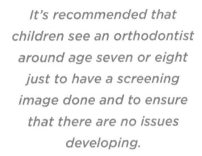

It's recommended that children see an orthodontist around age seven or eight just to have a screening image done and to ensure that there are no issues developing.

- **A regular dental appointment vs. an orthodontic appointment**

During a dental appointment, the first person you meet with is a hygienist, who gives your teeth a good deep cleaning and checks for cavities. Then the dentist comes in and does his exam, confirming any cavities found and gauging your overall oral health by checking your gums, teeth, and mouth for signs of disease or other conditions. During a dental visit, you may have some x-rays done, get a filling, undergo cosmetic bonding, or even have your teeth whitened.

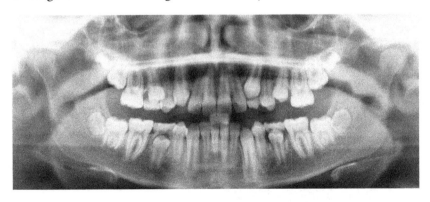

But if your teeth need straightening, that's when you see an orthodontist. An orthodontist, then, is a dentist who is also a specialist, focusing exclusively on the art and science of straightening teeth and jaws. A typical orthodontic case takes eighteen to twenty-four months to complete, and visits are typically spaced approximately six weeks apart. During this process, there are times when we'll see our patients more or less frequently than every six weeks, depending on what we're trying to accomplish.

• Care during orthodontic treatment

While we're working with patients to straighten their teeth, using appliances such as braces or Invisalign, it's incredibly important that patients see their dentists to keep their teeth clean and healthy before, during, and after treatment. Even though we're helping your teeth by straightening them out, that additional material in your mouth increases the risk of conditions such as swollen gums, decalcification, and—as with Sara's case at the beginning of this chapter—cavities developing around the braces.

In just a few months, cavities can form around braces if they're not well cleaned. Even without braces, if your teeth aren't straight and/or they're going through the process of being straightened, dentist appointments are vital to keeping those hard-to-reach areas clean. Adults are at an even greater risk for gum and periodontal (bone) issues, since they're more prone to buildup on the teeth. In any event, seeing a dentist is very important while you're undergoing orthodontic treatment!

While patients normally see their dentist twice a year, we prefer that our patients do so every four months during orthodontic treatment, particularly if they're at a higher risk for dental issues. Orthodontics is a significant investment of time, money, and effort, both for the orthodontist and the patient. The last thing we want interfering with a straight, beautiful smile is a preventable dental issue.

OUR DENTIST CONNECTION

Working with a patient's dentist during orthodontic treatment is so important to our practice that we're continually looking for ways to stay up-to-date and connected with dentists before, during, and after procedures. If a patient doesn't have a dentist when they see us, we refer them to someone we feel is the best fit for both their goals and their budget.

During the course of our patients' procedures, we check in regularly with their dentists to ensure that they're being seen and are receiving the necessary follow up. It is good for us as orthodontists to know that our patients are staying healthy, and it's good for the dentists because they get to see their patients more regularly and they can diagnose and treat any problems in the process early on.

After treatment, we offer referrals for any needed or desired follow-up work, as this is usually the best time to have any needed dental work, such as crowns, cosmetic bonding, dental implants, or veneers, done. This is because dental work, out of necessity, is built to your current bite. If you want to have the strongest, most ideal setup for your teeth, then it's best to have dental work done when your bite is as close to ideal as possible. The results will leave your teeth functioning and looking that much better.

A patient of ours, Viviane, found this out for herself when she came to us with a concern about some recent cosmetic dental work. At twenty-eight years old, Viviane was a beautiful young woman whose front teeth had been visibly crowded for most of her life. Her parents couldn't afford orthodontics, and even though she found a job after college and was able to afford the treatment, she decided to put it off, thinking that braces would hurt her chances for career advancement by making her look too young.

Before she knew it, it was six months before her wedding day. Instead of going through orthodontics, she saw a cosmetic dentist who convinced her that she could give her the perfect smile. Viviane had veneers (porcelain coverings) and bonding done on her upper front teeth, which vastly improved her smile, but left her with the feeling that something wasn't quite right with her bite.

When she finally made it to our practice, it was apparent that the cosmetic dentist had done the best she could to mask Viviane's crowding. Some of the teeth were cut down and others bulked out to give them the appearance of being straight. We were confident that we could give her the smile of her dreams—only this time it was going to be done to the standards of ideal dentistry, coordinating orthodontics with cosmetics.

The first step was to remove the bondings and veneers, so we could see the true position of her teeth. After that, she went through about twelve months of orthodontics to get her teeth in the ideal position. Prior to removing her braces, we made sure her cosmetic dentist was completely satisfied with the position of her teeth. With her approval, Viviane had new veneers placed, and the result was an amazing smile. She couldn't have been happier, and it was a rewarding day for all of us.

ORTHODONTICS IS A SPECIALTY; DON'T DO IT ON YOUR OWN!

Even though there's record of the ancient Greeks and even ancient Egyptians doing rudimentary orthodontic procedures, orthodontics didn't become a specialty until 1901.

Specifically, orthodontics is a specialization within dentistry that focuses on issues with the teeth and jaw." To become an orthodontist, you need to graduate from dental school and then go through an additional two to three years in an accredited orthodontics residency program. This is because straightening teeth is an incredibly complex and intricate process that takes years to understand and even longer to learn how to practice, which is why, when we graduate from an orthodontic residency program, we're considered specialists. We spend years exclusively studying the art and science of moving teeth through bone, and how that movement corresponds with the surrounding dental structures, jaw anatomy, and function. Most importantly, we exclusively practice orthodontics for eight to ten hours a day, five to six days a week, which means that seeing an orthodontist means seeing someone who is at the top of the game and is among the best in the field.

A general dentist can provide all aspects of dental care. While it is true that there are dentists who can provide orthodontic treatment, and some may do an excellent job, in general you are going to receive superior service by seeing an orthodontic specialist. While we don't mean any disrespect to our dental colleagues who do provide orthodontic services, they are often not equipped to practice it, nor do they have the same level of training as orthodontists.

When we do run into people who tell us that they decided to do orthodontics with their general dentist, the most common reasons they give us for doing so are:

- It was convenient to see their regular dentist.

- They don't want to insult their dentist by asking for an orthodontic referral.

- They thought they couldn't afford to see an orthodontist.

While we completely understand this mind-set, we often try to gently reframe the situation from a slightly different point of view.

For example, if your medical doctor were to recommend that you have your eyes checked for a possible procedure, you wouldn't ask him or her to do the exam. Instead, you'd go see an ophthalmologist (eye specialist). We all value our vision, so we see someone who specializes in eyes when they need care. Having your teeth straightened really is no different. You want to see a specialist, someone who is top of the field, so that you get the best esthetic and functional result for your smile.

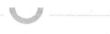

You want to see a specialist, someone who is top of the field, so that you get the best esthetic and functional result for your smile.

IT'S NOT THE TOOLS; IT'S THE SKILL OF THE PERSON USING THEM

We are very fortunate with respect to our area of health care that, while dentistry can improve your overall dental health, orthodontics is often elective and done primarily for esthetic reasons. In fact, there's a common perception that orthodontics is a commodity; that braces, for instance, are just put on your teeth and everything magically aligns. This perception is even more prevalent with Invisalign, with many people believing that as long as they're getting Invisalign, they're getting the same results no matter where they go to get it.

This couldn't be further from the truth. Braces and Invisalign are just tools to align your teeth. Invisalign is an excellent product, but successful results depend on the skills and expertise of the doctors *behind* those tools.

Seeing a specialist is an investment, but it's your long-term health and well-being—or the health and well-being of a loved one—that's on the line. Your body is with you for a lifetime; don't you want to keep it in the best working order possible for as long as you can?

When it comes to paying for that treatment, our fees are very reasonable for the level of specialty care you are getting. We also never want fees to be the reason someone does not have orthodontic treatment with us. That is why we're also very flexible when it comes to considering the overall and incremental costs that affect our patients. When you consider that our payment plans can be as low as $99 per month, well below the cost of a common smartphone plan, orthodontic procedures at our office really are affordable!

THE DAMAGE DONE BY DO-IT-YOURSELF ORTHODONTICS

What we don't want happening is for your condition to go untreated or, perhaps worse, for you to take matters into your own hands and attempt to fix it on your own. There is a new trend called "DIY orthodontics" in which people attempt at-home treatments, often relying on "advice" they find on the Internet. This disturbing trend has resulted in more injuries and harm than we can count, with patients just as likely to wind up in the ER as they are to visit our treatment rooms to fix the damage they've done. From rubber bands tied around molars to dental floss tied around incisors, it's safe to say we've pretty much seen it all—which is why trying to straighten your own teeth without seeing either a dentist or an orthodontist is a remarkably bad idea.

Another trend that has emerged in recent years is the home-aligner treatment. This involves either taking your own impressions or going to a scanning center to get started, then simply sitting back and waiting for your aligners to arrive in the mail. While the theory behind this is good, and the price cannot be matched, the reality is that orthodontics is not that simple. As of this writing (2018), there are five different companies in the US providing this service. The reality is that without a doctor watching your case, there is simply no reliable way to know that you're getting the best results. After treating thousands of cases with aligners, we can say with confidence that just because an aligner company tells you a tooth is going to move in a certain way, that doesn't mean it will.

Of course, we believe there is a market for this type of treatment; it can be used for minor DIY jobs in the same way that you don't have to be a contractor to do minor repairs around your house. Over time, too, this new trend may find a place in the overall orthodontic community, but there still a lot of work to be done before this type of treatment option finds a permanent place in our field.

One patient of ours found this out the hard way. As a young woman living in Manhattan, she frequently took the subway to work and often saw ads for a popular at-home tooth-straightening kit that promised to straighten teeth for a fraction of the cost of braces. She investigated it, and the price seemed like a no-brainer, so she ordered the kit. Everything seemed to be going fine until about eight weeks into her treatment, when she started feeling pain in her left-front tooth. Not knowing any better, she just assumed it was normal and kept going. Four weeks after that, she also noticed some swelling around the tooth but still thought it wasn't anything to be concerned about. A few weeks later, she woke up in significant pain with a great deal of swelling and had to see an endodontist for an emergency root canal. In the end, she missed several days of work and had to go through a week-long cycle of antibiotics to treat the condition.

The problem was that the tooth had suffered trauma at some point in the past and never received treatment—a condition that an orthodontist would have noticed and accounted for, if only she'd seen one. In going the DIY route, however, not only was she out the cost of the kit, but the attempt also cost her several days of work, several weeks of pain, and the cost of an emergency root canal. And she *still* needed to see an orthodontist to repair the damage done.

While this is a more dramatic scenario than most, it's unfortunately not unusual. With DIY tooth straightening, you miss out on the benefit of a doctor's diagnosis, which will not only evaluate where your teeth need to go to achieve an ideal position, but it will also tell you how they got to where they are in the first place. The diagnostic imaging that an orthodontist does before any tooth-straightening procedure accounts for past and current conditions of the teeth, jaws, and entire craniofacial area before making the best and most informed recommendation for moving forward. This part of the process is so vital that, if we no longer had access to it, we would say with confidence that we could no longer effectively do orthodontics.

On the surface, the DIY programs sold on the price difference of buying a kit versus seeing an orthodontist may look appealing. We get that. As a consumer, the price is appealing, as is the fact that you don't need to make time to go see an orthodontist to get your teeth straightened. But keep in mind that as you're going through treatment, with every visit we're reevaluating your teeth to make sure everything is doing what it should be—and sometimes, it's not. Sometimes we need to add in the use of rubber bands, or change how the rubber bands are being worn, or do something else to alter the amount or direction of force so that the teeth ultimately come into their ideal position.

You don't buy a DIY pacemaker for a heart condition, or go see a general practitioner for heart surgery, right? The same goes with the intricacies of tooth movement; it's something that needs to be done thoroughly and accurately by a professional.

A good orthodontist is going to guide your teeth in the right way and provide you with a deeper understanding of what to expect from your orthodontic treatment.

CHAPTER 2

Phase One Treatment

By Seth Newman, DDS

"So, what brings you in?"

This is the first question we usually ask after we introduce ourselves during an office visit. Today, I was asking this to a seven-year-old girl named Kristen who'd come in with her mom. The girl was sitting with her back tucked into the clinical chair, looking around the room with wide eyes. Her mom was smiling but looked a little nervous, which was to be expected. Some people come to an orthodontist just to be reassured that everything is well and good with their oral development, but more often than not, they're visiting us because something doesn't seem quite right.

For young patients like Kristen, the reason they're in is usually one of two things: either their dentist saw an issue that he or she wanted an orthodontist to take a look at, or the parents took a look in their child's mouth and thought that it looked off—crowded teeth, for instance, or evidence of an overbite or underbite.

In this case, it was a dentist referral.

"She thought we should come in and get a screening x-ray, just to make sure her adult teeth are coming in the way they should," said the girl's mom.

I looked down at Kristen, who gave me a big, gap-toothed grin.

"Her bottom two front teeth are loose, but the new ones are already coming in. Is that normal?" the mom added.

"I see," I said, smiling back. "That's actually a very common occurrence, but it always helps to make sure everything is doing what it should, especially at this age, when we can catch it early."

I sat down and pulled my chair up next to Kristen.

Before we do anything with our patients, regardless of age, we make sure they're comfortable first. With kids, we'll introduce ourselves and then talk about something fun, like the outfit they're wearing, what they think of school, or how they're enjoying summer vacation or winter break.

"So what grade are you going into?" I asked her.

Kristen smiled again and held up two shy fingers.

"Second grade!" I said. "Wow, I would have thought you were going into high school."

She laughed. "No, I'm only seven!"

"Seven is a great age to see an orthodontist," I told her. "Do you know what we do here?"

She shook her head.

"Well, it's our job to make sure your teeth are straight and that your bite—the way your teeth fit together—is the best bite you could possibly have," I explained.

She nodded.

"Is it okay if I look at your teeth?" I asked. "You can look along with me, too, if you like. Here," I said, handing her a mirror. "Now you can watch and see all the things I see."

"Thanks!" She said, opening her mouth wide and apparently doing her best to spot her tonsils.

With all our patients, we make it a point not to talk in complex technical terms during their visit. We want them to understand exactly what's going on, and it doesn't help anyone if we use confusing medical jargon.

In Kristen's situation, I could have said this was a simple case of lingually erupting mandibular incisors, but instead, I said to her, "So your mom tells me you have shark teeth."

"Shark teeth!" she said, laughing and shaking her head. "I'm definitely not a shark."

"No," I said. "But when you get new teeth growing in behind your old ones, it can look like shark teeth, because sharks have all those rows of teeth in their mouths, right? In fact, shark teeth happen a lot with kids your age."

I turned to the computer screen next to Kristen's chair and pulled up a case image of a child who had come in with "shark teeth" several months earlier.

"This little boy came in with shark teeth on four different teeth, if you can believe that," I told her.

"What happened to him?" she asked.

I pulled up the next image, which showed the boy smiling, his four adult teeth almost completely grown in.

"He got new teeth!" I said. "But first, his baby teeth had to fall out, and we had to take an x-ray to make sure his new teeth were coming in straight."

I pulled up an image of the boy's x-rays.

"We're going to take the same picture of your teeth, just to make sure everything is coming in the way it should, too," I told her.

She looked concerned. "Will it hurt?" she asked.

"Not at all," I said. "It's just a picture, and you even get to wear a special outfit when we take it," I said, meaning the protective lead vest we drape over our patient's chests before imaging.

This part of the process—showing patients images of cases similar to their own—is something we do with everyone. We have a bank of thousands of images, and most of the time we know which cases are appropriate to show for which kind of problems they have. I have my go-to cases for classic overbites and underbites, for instance, and in a lot of cases we also have an animation of the treatment—created by Dolphin Imaging—that shows exactly how the teeth will move over the course of the treatment.

This easing-in process, of providing as much clear and straight-forward information as possible up-front and showing patients how the same treatment has helped other real patients, is incredibly helpful in reducing anxiety and, in some cases, even gets the patient excited about what we're going to do next.

COMMON QUESTIONS FROM THE PARENTS

Every patient is unique, but there are a handful of questions that parents will often ask us during their child's first visit.

"Do they really need it?"

"Is it too early to be doing this?"

"Shouldn't we wait? He still has his baby teeth."

If the child is presenting with a jaw issue, such as a crossbite (when some or many of the upper teeth are sitting inside the lower teeth), overbite (when the top teeth vertically overlap the bottom teeth more than just a couple of millimeters), inadequate room for the developing permanent teeth, or underbite (also known as a crossbite in the front), the answer to all of these questions is that *now* is the best time to begin treatment.

Orthodontists call this "Phase One Treatment" or "Interceptive Orthodontic Therapy," and instead of focusing on the teeth, it's directed at changing jaw growth. For growing children, the earlier you fix a jaw issue, the more stable the results and subsequent jaw growth patterns are going to be. You can imagine how much growth a seven-year-old has ahead of her compared with a twelve- or thirteen-year-old. That window of opportunity, when the jaws are more malleable, is the best time to guide the jaws into a correct growth pattern.

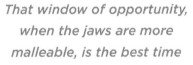

That window of opportunity, when the jaws are more malleable, is the best time to guide the jaws into a correct growth pattern.

We call this "phase one" treatment because we have found that nearly three out of four children who undergo it need a second phase of treatment when all their permanent teeth are in. In the first phase we correct the jaw issue to make room for the teeth that are still developing, but that doesn't mean that the new permanent teeth are going to come in straight. So, when the other teeth grow in, if they're still destined to grow in crooked or at an angle or rotated, then we need to address that in the second phase.

While directed at jaw discrepancies, Phase one treatment is also designed to make room for a child's developing dentition. As orthodontists, we can look at a seven- or eight-year-old child and successfully predict with a clinical exam, x-rays, models, and pictures (also referred to as "records") whether the young patient will have room for all of his or her developing teeth. If not, then we need to address the issue now, as that growth pattern is not going to change. Phase one treatment can develop kids' jaws so that they have enough room for all the adult teeth. Kids who need phase one treatment but do not have the benefit of treatment may likely need extractions or will have to deal with impacted teeth. If we address the condition with interceptive Phase One treatment, however, we can make room for those developing teeth, enhance the dental arches, and avoid unnecessary impactions or extractions.

Every now and then we get lucky and an eleven- or twelve-year-old patient's teeth come in straight, or they only need very minor adjustments, which means phase two treatment is up to the parents, who can decide how ideal they want their kids teeth to be. We are biased and want everyone to have ideal teeth so, if you ask us, we are usually going to recommend the phase two, but we will also give an honest opinion if we feel it is not necessary. However, most of the time jaw issues also mean that the teeth are going to need some help coming into an ideal bite. Just because we fixed the jaw issue, or made room for the adult teeth, does not mean that they will come in aligned.

As a parent with three children, one of whom has already completed phase one treatment and another who is in the midst of it, I can certainly understand that some parents may have reservations about the treatment. They often worry that their child is too young or immature or may not be able to tolerate treatment. But from my own experience and from working with so many other kids this same age, I've found phase one patients to be some of the best patients I've ever worked with. In fact:

1. **Young kids tolerate with ease what adults do not, and they are more resilient than we often give them credit for.** Appliances such as palatal expanders, for instance, will certainly slow down an adult but not an eight-year-old. Within a few days, young children are usually functioning like normal and give little thought to the appliance in their mouth.

2. **They follow instructions.** When we need a youngster to help fix an overbite with elastics, they really follow the instructions and make us look like rock stars. That same child, grown into an adolescent, would likely be much less compliant and take twice as much effort for half as much result.

3. **Those who are the most apprehensive and fearful of the process quickly lose their anxiety after a handful of visits.** They quickly realize that we're not going to hurt them and that coming to the orthodontist can be fun. It's not uncommon for young patients to need a parent's assistance to have any treatment done. Sometimes it's as simple as a hand to hold, and while there may be some initial tears, these patients often turn around in only a few short visits. This new confidence can be a real source of pride for both the orthodontist and the parents.

How Does the Position of Baby Teeth Affect How the Permanent Teeth Grow In?

The position of the erupting permanent teeth is dictated more by the jaw than by the position of the baby teeth they're replacing. Ideally, baby teeth are spaced out in the jaws, which allows room for the permanent teeth to grow in. Sometimes, however, a baby tooth may take too long to fall out, such as we saw with Kristen, where the adult tooth was forced to erupt into a displaced "shark-tooth" position.

If a baby tooth falls out too early, it can affect the direction of growth of the adult tooth underneath. Baby teeth are often the guiding track for the adult teeth when they come into the mouth, and it is that development of the adult tooth that ultimately forces out the baby tooth. Additionally, an adult tooth may come in at a slight angle, either due to a baby tooth not falling out soon enough or because it started growing down a less-than-ideal path.

The position of the baby teeth can have an influence on where the adult teeth will erupt. However, it does not tell the whole story, which is why getting a screening x-ray just after the baby teeth start to fall out can be helpful in addressing tooth issues as soon as possible.

Can Thumb Sucking Affect My Child's Bite?

The most common habit we see that affects tooth position is thumb sucking. When a kid sucks his or her thumb, it does three things:

1. The thumb pushes the lower teeth in and presses the upper teeth out.

2. The inward suction can influence the jaws to grow in more narrowly.

3. The top and bottom teeth in the front do not meet, causing what we call an "open bite." This is when there is a significant opening between the upper and lower teeth. This is the opposite of an overbite, where there is excessive vertical overlapping of the lower and upper front teeth.

There is a common belief that the jaws can't move, but they do—probably more so than any other part of your body, based on the pressures that are being put on them. So, if a child has his or her thumb in her mouth several hours a day, it's going to have an impact.

Another habit called lip biting or lip sucking, in which the child sticks her lip between her top and bottom teeth and squeezes them together, can also have a negative impact as this action pushes out on the upper teeth.

In these cases, as is the case with any oral habit, the sooner the habit can be stopped, the better. And if you don't stop the habit before you correct the teeth, then the teeth will likely revert to the same bad bite.

At What Age Does Thumb Sucking Become a Problem?

Parents will often ask us this question and the answer really depends on the severity of the habit. Is the child sucking his or her thumb only while sleeping, or is he or she constantly walking around with finger in mouth? Generally, if the habit is stopped prior to losing the first baby teeth and before the adult teeth grow in (which tends to begin around age six), the impacts of the habit can sometimes naturally reverse themselves. If the habit continues once the adult teeth are present, however, it is best to seek some interventional therapy to correct it. My own son, Alex, used a pacifier until he was close to three years old, and I remember being alarmed by the fact that he developed an open bite. When it was finally time to kick the pacifier habit—and in only a few short months his open bite was gone.

Julie was one of my first thumb-sucking patients. She was only about seven years old, but if you heard her talk you would have thought she was seventeen. She was extremely smart, a keen negotiator, and had a severe thumb habit that had caused a significant open bite. Every time she came in, we would discuss this habit and she would debate with me about why it wasn't that big a problem. Our discussions felt like a model Congress.

When she finally conceded, her phase one treatment took about one year to finish. I was pleased with the orthodontic result, but deep down, I think I was prouder of my debating win.

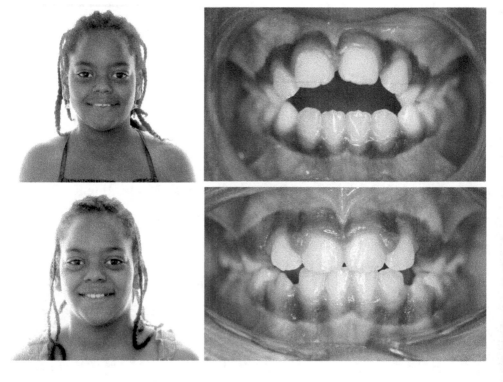

Julie continued to come in for her phase one follow-ups for a time, but somewhere along the line she stopped. The next time I saw her, she was twelve years old and smarter than ever ... but her open bite was back and as big as ever.

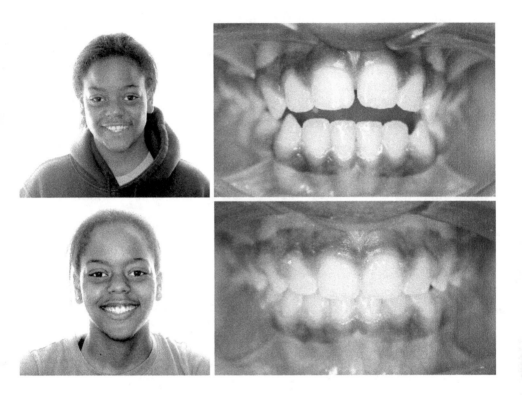

It was a significant blow to my ego, and I felt a little defeated that my argument against thumb sucking hadn't stuck. We talked about it and Julie admitted that she'd gone back to her old habits, and deep down she knew that her teeth turned out the way they were because of it. Back into braces she went, and eighteen months later, she came out of them with amazing results.

After that process, Julie and I both understood that a habit will always win. Even if orthodontics fixes a situation for a period of time, if the bad habit persists, the teeth will eventually shift again.

This is why, as orthodontists, we're not interested in simply treating symptoms, but also in properly diagnosing and addressing the problem's root cause.

How Can I Tell if My Child has Jaw Issues?

Most parents can just tell by looking. You don't need a degree in orthodontics to see if something just doesn't look right. Jaw discrepancies such as crossbite, overbite, and underbite, aren't just tooth-related: they can be seen by evaluating the position of the jaw and often by the developing shape of a child's face. If a child has an overbite, for instance, you can look at his or her profile and see that the upper jaw is more forward than the lower jaw, giving a convex appearance.

Crossbites (when the upper teeth are sitting inside of the lower teeth) can also be spotted by a parent just by asking the child to bite his or her teeth together and observing how the teeth fit.

Jaw discrepancies can be caused by a lot of things, such as bad oral habits, but more often than not, they're genetic.

In my experience, most parents are astute enough to know what is normal and what is not. They usually are not going to diagnose a problem, but they know enough to take their children to someone who can. We applaud these parents because they are the ones most likely to become our partners and cheerleaders in helping their children—our patients—comply with treatment.

How Are Jaw Issues Treated in Phase One?

It's exciting for us when we see young patients specifically for a jaw discrepancy, because it means that our referring doctors were keeping an extra sharp eye out for the condition. Between the ages of seven and nine is the ideal time to treat these conditions, as children this age have so much more growth ahead of them.

Crossbites are the most common jaw discrepancy we see in young patients, and treatment typically involves a palate expander in the upper jaw. This is almost always followed by fixed appliances, which we call "mini braces," to align the upper and lower adult teeth. By "mini," we don't mean "small," but rather that we're only placing braces on the adult teeth instead of all the teeth (though there are some cases where we may place braces on baby teeth, as well). Typically, this means braces on the first four adult teeth and the back molars.

The length of treatment is usually between twelve and eighteen months to get everything aligned, after which we give them a retainer to wear until the adult teeth have grown in.

For significant overbites and underbites, we have several orthodontic appliances that we can fit younger patients with, and most of the time they're very good at keeping up with them. Eight- or nine-year-old kids are often much more willing to wear rubber bands or be compliant with other devices when they're told, as opposed to twelve- or thirteen-year-olds—which is another reason starting treatment at a young age is better.

With all our younger patients, we recommend using fixed appliances (braces), as opposed to removable ones (retainers and night guards), mainly because you can't lose the fixed ones. With young kids especially, it's so easy for them to lose or break an appliance, or not wear it consistently. My son Alex, on whom I did a phase one treatment and who is now using a retainer, once forgot to pack his retainer for a family vacation, so for a week and a half he wasn't wearing it. That's why we recommend fixed appliances; when they're cemented in the mouth, there's nowhere for them to go, and only the orthodontist can remove them.

Can Orthodontic Treatment Affect My Child's Self-Esteem?

Children are inherently self-conscious—even more so as they get into middle and high school, which is another reason why we try to do what we can at an early age. Once they complete treatment, the confidence boost is significant.

For instance, we had a nine-year-old girl named Daisy who came in because she hated the spaces between her front teeth. We spoke with her about treatment options, and she agreed to have braces put on. Even before the gaps started closing, her mother pulled me aside and told me how much more confident her daughter was simply because she knew something was being done about her teeth. At that age, a lot of kids think that getting braces is cool, and she was proud to wear them. That alone helped to boost her self-esteem.

Will Early Treatment Prevent My Child from Needing Major Procedures Later in Life?

We tell all our Phase One patients that they should assume they are going to need Phase Two treatment when they're older, as the focus of Phase One is on jaw discrepancies and making sure that emerging teeth have enough room to grow in.

The typical Phase One patient has an average of twelve baby teeth and the same number of developing adult teeth, so if those adult teeth do not come in straight, Phase Two treatment will be needed to set them on the right path for an ideal bite. When there are significant jaw issues, such as a large overbite, a child who needs 100 percent correction may get 60 to 70 percent of the way there during phase one, and the remaining 30 percent can be handled during adolescence with phase two, or comprehensive orthodontics. However, if that same individual grows into adulthood without correcting his or her bite, we sometimes cannot get the full correction that would have been possible had interceptive phase one therapy taken place.

Even if a genetic jaw discrepancy led to the need for jaw surgery in adulthood, patients would still benefit from early treatment. Let's say a hypothetical patient had a 12 mm overbite without early treatment (orthodontics is a "millimeter profession," so 12 mm is a lot to us)—but *with* treatment, that same overbite was only 6 mm. Since orthodontics is a "millimeter profession," that patient would still need surgical therapy as an adult—but the magnitude of the surgical movements could be decreased dramatically, thereby decreasing the trauma associated with surgery. Plus, it would give us a shot at a much better outcome.

Phase one treatment is also important when making room for a child's developing teeth. If a child has no room for the adult teeth to come in, a phase one treatment to widen the jaws can prevent the need for extractions later on.

Take Sergio's case. At the age of seven, he came to us with such a bad overbite that he couldn't close his lips, and his front teeth stuck out like a chipmunk—which was the nickname his brothers and sisters gave him. The name-calling was bad enough, but Sergio was also active in sports, which meant his teeth were that much more at risk of being broken or knocked out.

We did a phase one treatment to expand his jaw and begin the process of moving and positioning his teeth back into his mouth, followed by a phase two to straighten them and complete treatment. Over the years, we were able to guide everything into a position that corrected his overbite and gave him ideal teeth. By the age of twelve, he got his braces off, and not only was his jaw corrected, he was getting compliments all the time on how nice his smile was. If he hadn't undergone that treatment early on, there's no way we could have gotten his teeth into such an ideal position. Fortunately, we caught him at just the right age when we were able to modify his growth and guide everything to where it needed to go.

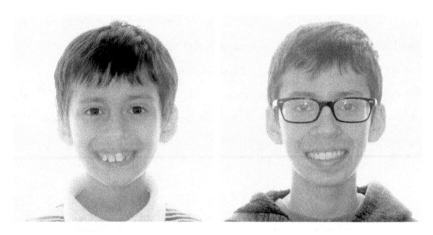

What Are My Responsibilities as a Parent during My Child's Treatment?

Phase one, or any other orthodontic treatment for children, is always going to be a hands-on experience for the parents. As a mom or dad, one of the most important things you need to do is make sure your child is brushing well—and if he or she has braces, brushing underneath, over, and around them every day. Braces should also be checked daily to make sure nothing is broken or poking the child in the mouth.

Another key to successful orthodontics may seem obvious, but is incredibly important to your child's progress, and that is coming in regularly for scheduled appointments. We understand that parents and kids today lead incredibly busy lives between family responsibilities, school, sports, etc. But, unfortunately, things happen—or, as we like to say in orthodontics, "shift happens"—when patients don't come in for their regular appointments for several months.

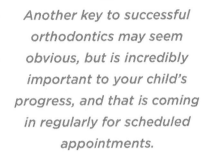

Another key to successful orthodontics may seem obvious, but is incredibly important to your child's progress, and that is coming in regularly for scheduled appointments.

For instance, if your child has a palate expander, the appliance needs to be adjusted regularly, which means you'll have to turn it at home, and we'll need to do monitor the progress in the office. Our standard protocol is to turn the expander as little as one to two turns per week to as often as once every other day. This of course, all depends on the individual patient's needs, the type of appliance, the timeline for treatment, and our overall goals. Ultimately, we believe that slow and steady wins the race.

When young patients complete the initial phase of orthodontics, we usually ask that they wear their retainer only at night. This gives them a predictable schedule to follow and minimizes the chances that they'll lose their retainer at school or anywhere else throughout the day.

It should be noted that retention wear in patients who have had phase one treatment is usually temporary, as opposed to patients who have undergone comprehensive or full orthodontics, in which case we like to say, "Retention Is for Life." This is because typical patients who complete phase one treatment may or may not lose their baby teeth soon after that treatment is completed. Once baby teeth start to fall out, we ask our phase one patients to stop wearing their retainers, giving them a "Retainer Holiday" until their adult teeth come in. Wearing the retainer too long can interfere with the eruption of the adult teeth. That is why we like to see our patients who are in phase one retention every two to three months. Once all the adult teeth grow in, we can either make them a new retainer or begin phase two treatment if needed.

Phase one treatment can have dramatic results when needed. It can really have a huge impact on your child's growth and development. Not every child needs it, but those who do can experience significant beneficial changes. Just remember that, as a parent, the more active you are in your child's orthodontic treatment, the better the results.

CHAPTER 3

Adolescent Orthodontics

By Efstathios Giannoutsos, DDS

Steven and Megan couldn't have been more different from each other. Megan, twelve years old, was one the brightest and most inquisitive patients I'd ever met, while her thirteen-year-old brother, Steven, was one of the shyest and most reserved.

I could see the difference between the two even before we began our consultation. Megan was walking around the room, peering at the pictures, and checking out the dental models of different braces on my desk, while Steven stood next to his dad, hands in his pockets, staring at his shoes.

Every patient has a different level of comfort the first time they come in. While some are ready to go, others have some reservations. Those are the patients we need to ease into orthodontics by spending lots of time talking so that they completely understand what orthodontics can do before any work is done. When people understand that no procedure is going to happen that first day (unless they want it to), it immediately puts them in a calmer state of mind and makes them more willing to talk about treatment options.

With adolescent patients, we begin our consultation the same way every time, starting with broad questions and then gradually working our way toward the education part.

"So, what brings you in today?" I asked them.

Megan was the first to speak up. "Doc thinks we have some jaw problems you could help us out with. Overbite for me, and Steven has a crossbite." She paused, saw an expander on the table, and picked it up to start fiddling with it. "What does this do?"

"That is what we use to widen jaws for people with cross..." I stopped because Steven suddenly looked a little pale.

"You know what?" I said, "I think we need to sit down and just talk about what it is that orthodontists do—what you can expect from your visits here—and then I can answer any questions you have."

Megan nodded and took a seat. I looked up at Steven and his dad, and Dad gave me the nod to go ahead while Steven stayed where he was.

I picked up two patient mirrors and handed one to Megan and placed the other on a side table next to Steven.

"Megan, would you like to help me out for a minute?" I asked.

"Sure!" she said.

"Okay, I'm not going to touch your teeth, but I'd like to talk with you about what's going on in your mouth," I said. "Could you open your mouth and then hold up the mirror, so you can watch while I point them out?" I gave her a mirror, which she was able to use to follow the things I was pointing out about her teeth.

For the next few minutes, I pointed out to Megan—with Steven half watching from the corner—what was an adult tooth, what was a baby tooth, what was coming in the wrong way, what was rotated, where there were spaces, and just a few other general observations. I noted that her twelve-year molars were coming in nicely and pointed out that not everyone gets their twelve-year molars at exactly twelve years old; sometimes it takes until they turn thirteen or even fourteen for them to appear. She looked pleased.

Next, I asked Megan to put down the mirror and I pulled up a video clip of a standard overbite treatment.

"Your dentist was correct, Megan," I said. "You do appear to have an overbite, just like the patient in this video. To treat it, you're probably going to need to wear braces, and this will show you exactly how we do that."

Afterward, Megan asked about twenty questions, including what her color options would be on the elastic bands, and how soon we could get started. Steven, on the other hand, still hadn't said a word.

"Do you have any questions, Steven?" I asked.

He hesitated a moment, then asked, "When do you do the drilling part?"

I wasn't surprised; it was a very common question.

"We don't do that here," I said reassuringly. "Orthodontics is more about the long-term movement of teeth and jaws. Just about everything we do is gradual and involves very little to no pain—and that 'little' pain is usually more of a soreness than anything else; like the kind of sore you feel after a tough sports practice. Do you play a sport?" I asked.

He nodded. "Soccer," he said.

"There you go," I said. "It's like how you feel the morning after a big match."

Steven nodded but didn't say anything else.

"I'll tell you what," I said. "Megan, let's go ahead and do your records, and get you scheduled to put your braces on. Steven, how about we set up one more consultation—just me, you, and your dad; no procedures involved. Sound good?"

We'll often suggest a second consultation for particularly anxious patients, which Steven certainly was. Megan took off with Jiselle, one of our orthodontic assistants, to get her imaging (x-rays and pictures) done, and I asked Steven if he wanted to watch.

"No," he said, and then asked, "What are they doing an x-ray for?"

"Every patient, regardless of age, requires the same set of orthodontic records to be evaluated for proper diagnosis and treatment planning," I explained. "Those records consist of pictures of the face, teeth, and jaws together, and a scan of the mouth so detailed that it allows us to 3-D print your teeth and jaws, if we need to. The x-rays—there are two of them, called a panoramic x-ray and a cephalometric x-ray—let us see how many teeth you have, what direction they're growing, and how your jaws are developing. Occasionally we also do a supplemental x-ray, but that's only if we see some asymmetries in your skeletal structure that we want to check on."

"Okay," he said. "So, no drilling, huh?"

"Not in the slightest," I said. "There is an instrument that looks a little like a drill that we use to polish teeth, but I'll show that to you at our next meeting. No pain, just a fine polished finish at the end on your enamel."

The next meeting with Steven went well. Without his sister there, he sat down next to his dad and even opened his mouth, so I could do the same walkthrough I'd done with his sister. I showed him our digital scanner. When I explained to Steven that the scanner takes thousands of pictures a second to build a 3-D model of your teeth he thought that was pretty cool. He told me that the building of the scan of someone's teeth was like when he built things in Minecraft, his favorite video game, and I could see he was warming up to our office. We then watched a video on a standard crossbite treatment and I showed him a model of braces. He was finally ready to look at and hold the expander his sister had been playing with during their first visit, and I demonstrated how it fit on the molars and how the famous and dreaded "key" could be used to tighten it as often as needed.

By the end of it, we'd demystified the entire process and Steven was even willing to do his x-ray. It turned out he was also a great candidate for removable-aligner treatment with Invisalign after expander treatment, and when I told him that, it seemed to brighten him up.

"And I'll tell you what," I said. "We'll also send you your orthodontic simulation file, which we'll generate after we scan your teeth today. I'll email it to your mom and dad before our next appointment, so you can see exactly how we plan to move your teeth. Also, since you said you wanted to do Invisalign but you understand we must correct your crossbite first and wait for some teeth to come in, I can tell you about how many aligners you'll need after we do your expansion. You will also know where you may need any little bumps, also called attachments, that we use to help move your teeth. And if you need to just talk again without a procedure following it, we can do that, too. We'll take this as slowly as you need to so that you're as comfortable as you can be with the entire process."

REDUCING FEAR AND ANXIETY IN ADOLESCENT PATIENTS

For Megan, the idea of getting braces was fun. Many of our young patients are actually excited to get their braces on. They can't wait to get them on and think they are cool, especially when many of their friends start wearing them.

In these cases, we've found that the more information we can provide our young patients, the better. Just like a pilot can calm an anxious flyer by explaining how the plane is going to fly and what to expect regarding trip time and weather, we walk them through every step of the process, answering any questions they have along the way.

If they're still anxious, the next step we take is a gradual easing in to the treatment. For Steven's crossbite, for example, we may just start with the expander, letting him wear it for a few months before activating it and using the key to tighten it. If he was doing braces instead of Invisalign, we might start with just the top braces for a few months, then put the lower braces on and, a few months after that, take the expander out. We've learned that it's gradual changes like these that make the process more tolerable for anxious patients, tailoring it to their specific needs.

We also have our secret weapon we use when needed. This is our very highly skilled staff members who are almost like child whisperers. They spend some extra time with these patients and help ease them into the process of treatment.

Orthodontic offices, like any medical office, are inherently chaotic, so simply removing anxious patients from that environment and putting them in a private clinical room can reduce some of that intense anxiety.

For those who need a little extra tender loving care, like our special needs patients, we do a slow desensitization, letting them touch the devices we're going to put in their mouths, get comfortable with everything—possibly only doing an appointment where we introduce them to the braces, brackets, and wires without putting any of them on. Then we often take it slow but putting on a few braces in the beginning before we introduce a full set.

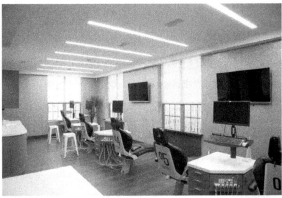

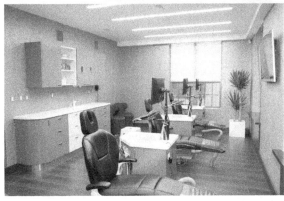

At the same time that we're easing these patients through the process, keeping things quiet and consistent, we're also encouraging in them the desire to join the masses. Most kids don't want to always go into the private clinical room—they want to join the group of kids in the open bay, or they want to join a sibling, who's already out there. With siblings like Megan and Steven, often they're sitting in the open bay together by month six, joking with each other, and so comfortable with the process that they're already bored with it, asking when they're going to be done.

WHAT DETERMINES THE TIMING OF ADOLESCENT ORTHODONTIC TREATMENT?

The first thing we look for in an adolescent patient's mouth is how many of the adult teeth have come in and how many baby teeth are remaining. The last few teeth to come in are typically the upper canines, the pre-molars, and the twelve-year molars, which, again, don't always come in at the age of twelve. If the patient has some baby teeth, we may encourage him or her to help us wiggle them out so we can guide the adult teeth in, or we might ask the general dentist to extract some select teeth in order to encourage the underlying adult teeth to grow in.

We'll also take the growth of the child's face into account, as certain changes just before or at the start of puberty can occur that will profoundly affect orthodontics. Because of this, we make note of certain characteristics and observe them for changes over the course of treatment, or we'll gauge those changes to determine the best time to start treatment and take advantage of that growth. Also—and this is not commonly mentioned—we look closely at both biological parents to take stock of their facial characteristics, providing us with very important bits of information in treating our young patients.

It's with adolescent orthodontics that the practice of orthodontics becomes more art than science. We have to gauge those things that need to be accomplished now, before growth ends, and those things that can be adjusted later, as well as those things that only nature can take care of at her own pace. Once a child is done with puberty, the suture in the upper jaw (that little separation of the two upper jaw bones) seals and there's no way to adjust it without surgical intervention—precisely what we're hoping to avoid. Sometimes this means having the child come in every six months or so, just watching the last few teeth as they come in, until it's the best time to start. Other times, we may be able to start right away. We may also wait a little more if the child is anxious and not ready to start, or if he or she is adamantly against braces and wants to wait for all of the adult teeth in order to do Invisalign.

What's important at the adolescent stage of development is that the patient and parents understand that this is a critical timeframe; we only have a handful of years to make changes that will span a lifetime.

PATIENT PATIENCE: HELPING ADOLESCENTS THROUGH THEIR ORTHODONTIC TREATMENT

One of the most important things we've learned about treating adolescents—and really any patients—is that we need to wait until they're ready, until they can understand that we're partners in the process. The days of the paternalistic "You have to do it because I told you so" practice is over. You can't just force treatment on a child. I've had a few young patients who have simply ripped the brackets off their teeth or crushed their retainers because they were forced into treatment. All this does is leave the parents embarrassed—they've incurred a cost, and the child has acted out and is upset. In such cases, we'd lose the partnership that is so necessary to successful treatment, and no one would be happy in the end.

In instances like those, we tell the parents that the action was no one's fault. Orthodontics is a feel-good profession, and if their son or daughter doesn't want to go through the process now, or if he or she needs a little bit of a break, then we can do that. It's better to pause momentarily and let the patient feel like he or she has a choice instead of trying to force it on anyone. All we ask is that the patient come in periodically for a checkup so we can make sure we're not missing a critical window. In fact, this slower easing in is often all that the child needs to feel comfortable with the process.

Over the years, I've found that my best adolescent patients are—you probably guessed it—the most cooperative ones.

Over the years, I've found that my best adolescent patients are—you probably guessed it—the most cooperative ones. Not only do they take excellent care of their braces but they follow directions to a tee, which makes us look like orthodontic super stars. Some of our best cooperators or partners don't necessarily want the treatment but are willing to go through with it and follow instructions so they can finish as soon as possible. And that's the key! Those kids that say, "What do I have to do to get these things off as soon as possible?" are the ones that break records on treatment completion. They can accomplish in mere months in what sometimes can take years in others. If we tell them to wear rubber bands, they'll wear them full time. They follow the food-avoidance rules, and ultimately, they wind up with the most profound changes in the least amount of time.

Orthodontic treatment is only as good as our patient's worst day in a given month, which is why we engage in what we call a "therapeutic contract" with our patients. This contract makes it clear that we're providing a service that our patients are aware is beneficial to them, and they've chosen to go through with. If they don't want to do it, we won't do it. Simple as that. Just as a physician may tell an overweight patient to eat right and exercise, unless the patient is willing to be partners in the process, the results won't be there. The same goes with orthodontics. If you're not willing to put the time and effort in, it's not going to work.

WHAT EXACTLY IS ADOLESCENT ORTHODONTIC TREATMENT?

If you close your eyes and picture someone in braces, most of us think of think of a young person, usually between the ages of eleven and thirteen. This traditionally has been the most common time for braces treatment, as it's the earliest point at which all the baby teeth are gone, and the adult teeth are growing in.

As orthodontists, we like to place braces as soon as those adult teeth are present. This gives us the opportunity to correct the root cause of a bad bite before kids hit that pubertal growth spurt, giving us the advantage of that growth and directing it in a favorable way to fix any orthodontic issues.

Overbites, underbites, crossbites, and open bites are all orthodontic terms you've likely heard before, and all these things, when there are discrepancies, can contribute to a bad bite. Most of our patients do not present with just tooth-crowding or spacing issues; usually there's a jaw discrepancy at play that needs to be encouraged into a better growth direction, and the sooner we start shaping that growth, the better.

Orthodontic treatment at this age usually consists of a full set of braces on the adult teeth, and any baby teeth remaining may be used as anchors to temporarily move the adult teeth.

WHEN DO WE NEED MORE THAN JUST BRACES?

It's not uncommon for other appliances, such as palatal expanders, to be used in conjunction with braces, and rubber bands are common in guiding the upper and lower teeth into a better fit.

Apart from expanders, the most common types of appliances that we use are:

- **Trans-Palatal Arches (TPA):** a permanent wire that arches across the top of the mouth and is fixed onto the first molars. It can be used to save space in the top arch or to use as an anchor for moving other teeth.

- **Lower Lingual Holding Arches (LLHA):** much like the TPA but for the lower jaw. The LLHA is fixed onto the first molars and arches against the back of the lower teeth (lingually). Its main use is to keep your lower molars from moving, though it may sometimes be used as an anchor to move other teeth.

- **Herbst/Forsus/MARA Appliances:** permanent devices that are fixed to the back of the teeth. They are designed to move the upper and lower jaws into harmony by restricting the upper-jaw growth and promoting a more horizontal lower-jaw growth.

- **Facemask:** to promote forward growth of the upper jaw.

- **Tongue Crib/habit appliance:** to prevent the placement of a thumb, the tongue, or the lips between the teeth.

- **Distalizers:** to move teeth back in the upper jaw to create space.

- **Turbos:** helps to lessen the severity and correct a deep overbite.

- **Accelerated Orthodontic Devices:** vibration technology that stimulates increased blood flow and tooth movements and can lessen treatment time.

- **Self-ligating braces:** reduce friction and can help severely crowded cases unravel faster.

RUBBER BANDS: THEY'RE NOT JUST FOR SNAPPING AT YOUR BROTHER

Without question, rubber bands are the most powerful auxiliaries that we ask our patients to use for the improvement of their overall results, minimization of treatment time, and for the optimization and control of the forces placed on the brace/wire/Invisalign system. The most common reason we are using elastics is for the improvement of the forward/backward (sagittal) relationship of the upper and lower jaws when viewed from the profile. Another major reason we use elastics is to improve the way the upper and lower teeth fit together. Braces can straighten their teeth in the respective jaws, but to get the jaws to where they are functioning in a harmonious fashion can sometimes only be effectively achieved through the use of rubber bands.

When adolescence and adults wear their rubber bands as instructed, we can achieve dramatic results. Overbites and under-bites get corrected, the teeth align faster than without them, and the fit between the upper and lower teeth is improved. When our patients are disciplined and follow the elastic regime, they make us look great. We as orthodontists often get super excited about this and tell them how wonderful they are doing. They, in turn, have a sense of pride and ownership in their orthodontic results, and continue to be compliant, and maximize the efficiency of their treatment.

There is a good reason why we get so excited when patients are effectively wearing the rubber bands. Unfortunately, for every patient who does wear them well, there are another one to two who does not. We can tell in a second if patients are really wearing them or not. Oftentimes, there will be little if any difference from the prior visit if they had not been worn effectively. These often make for some of the most interesting moments in our busy day. We have literally heard it all:

"Doc, I got to be honest, those things are bad for my social life," said ten-year-old Charlie.

"Dad, he totally would have never known, why did you have to tell him," said twelve-year-old Alex

"I tried wearing them, but every time I would chew gum, it would get stuck in the rubber bands," said thirteen-year-old Kaylee.

We see our patients sometimes for as little as ten minutes. Having them buy into the importance of elastic wear and be compliant with wearing them—oftentimes 24/7 for the next six weeks—is not without its challenges. That is why we understand when they have not been worn as instructed. We then try to do our best to educate and motivate our patients to understand the importance of elastics wear. Usually, with encouragement, this is largely effective. For those who cannot be convinced, we have "non-compliance appliances." We prefer to only use them when we cannot convince our patients to wear elastics, a.k.a. "rubber bands." They tend to be cumbersome and sometimes uncomfortable which is why we prefer to use elastics.

Many in our field believe that there is practically *no difference* in overall results achieved when we have a compliant young man or woman who uses elastics compared with someone fitted "non-compliance appliance."

WHAT ARE THE TREATMENT OPTIONS FOR ADOLESCENTS?

Technology dominates most aspects of our teen's lives, so why should their orthodontics be any different? Advances in orthodontics allow us to move teeth faster, with more precision, and more comfortably than ever before, with state-of-the-art options including Invisalign teen removable aligners, virtually invisible ceramic braces, and modern metal braces.

Metal Braces

Although these may look like standard metal braces, there's nothing traditional about them. Advancements in technology have made metal braces more efficient and more comfortable than ever before, with thin, customized arch wires running through laser cut, surgical-grade stainless steel brackets that have been bonded onto the surface of each tooth. Over time, these wires gently guide your child's teeth into their ideal position, resulting in that gorgeous smile.

Holding each of these arch wires in place is a very small rubber band (not to be confused with the rubber band we use to correct the bite and is attached between the two jaws) that kids can customize with a variety of colors! We can change these colors at every visit. If you or your child wants to sport a little Halloween spirit with black and orange, go for it! Changing colors is a relatively fast procedure, too. So, if your daughter wants to have her braces match her dress for an event, come on in. Our staff will be just as excited as she is to help color-coordinate her braces.

Clear (Ceramic) Braces

If you're seeking all the benefits of braces but also want amazing esthetics, clear braces are the way to go. Today's ceramic brackets are made from zirconium—the same material used to make fake diamonds—which renders them nearly invisible. They are so clear that you and your friends may forget that you are wearing them.

Just as with metal braces, ceramic brackets are glued onto the surface of each individual tooth, combining them with a thin, high-esthetic wire designed to blend in with your natural tooth color. The wire is then held in place with clear elastics so that they are virtually invisible, creating an overall discreet alternative to traditional metal.

Invisalign Teen-Removable Aligners

These aligners are specifically designed with the needs of our adolescent patients in mind. Customized to the growing mouths of teens, these clear, removable aligners are an invisible method of straightening teeth and, when worn properly, are just as effective as braces.

Additionally, the removable nature of the aligners allows teens to take them out for activities such as sports or playing musical instruments. Also, because they are removable, they can eat all the hard foods they want with no restrictions. Ideally, Invisalign teen aligners should be worn a minimum of twenty-two hours a day and are removed when eating and while brushing or flossing.

One of the nice features of the Invisalign teen product that differs from the regular Invisalign model is a little blue tab, which turns clear over time. This indicator tab allows us to see if our teen patients have been wearing the aligners for the prescribed amount of time.

Invisalign knows its teen population. That is why they have built in free replacement aligners in case of loss. Incidentally, we find our teen patients to be more compliant than some of the adults—probably because they are being threatened with wearing braces if the aligners don't work. Loss of aligners happens rarely, and it's usually our adult patients who do this!

The technological advancements with Invisalign Teen have been truly remarkable. We can accomplish things that were not predictably doable only a few years ago. Today, Invisalign and Invisalign teen can both achieve results as good as braces and include auxiliaries such as rubber bands to accomplish more complex movements that before were limited to fixed braces alone.

CHAPTER 4

Does Your Child Really Need Braces?

By Seth Newman, DDS

If you were to search online for the best age to take your child to an orthodontist, you would find that the official answer from the American Association of Orthodontics is that everyone should get an orthodontic screening at age seven. Why? It's at this age that orthodontists can tell if any developmental issues will become problems, and the sooner those issues can be addressed, the better.

Our patients often come to us for the first time because their dentist recommended it. This was exactly the case for eight-year-old John, whose mother brought him in at the urging of their family dentist. He'd noticed that John's back teeth appeared to be out of alignment, with the top teeth slipping inside the bottom teeth whenever he bit down.

"She called it a posterior crossbite," John's mom said as I looked at his mouth. John, who was holding up the patient mirror, so he could follow along, nodded.

"It looks like it," I said. "And I'm glad your dentist caught this. Dentists really are our first line of defense when it comes to keeping your bite as close to ideal as possible. It seems you do have a posterior crossbite and that you've created a functional shift, too."

"What's that?" said John, angling the mirror around in an attempt to find it.

"It has to do with the position of your jaw," I explained. "See, since your teeth weren't fitting together quite right in the back, you started moving your jaw to one side so that you could comfortably perform everyday functions, like chewing."

"I see," his mom said, frowning. "Could we have done anything to prevent those conditions—the crossbite and shift?"

I shook my head. "A crossbite is truly a skeletal or jaw discrepancy. It just means that the upper jaw is too narrow for the lower jaw, which is quite often a genetic condition. Think of it like a shoebox—if the lid is too small for the box, it just falls right into the box instead of fitting snugly on top, right? In this case, to make up for the small lid, John began shifting his lower jaw to the right or left so he could properly bite down on one side, which is why we call it a functional shift. This habit can result in uneven, or asymmetric, jaw function and uneven lower-jaw growth, which is why it's good that we're able to address this now. At eight years old, John is the perfect candidate for dentofacial orthopedics, which is a fancy way of saying that we can take advantage of this rapid growth stage through jaw-growth modification. Not treating these conditions now will only make these more difficult to treat later as his bone structure matures and hardens."

"How do you guide that growth, then? Braces?" his mom asked. "I had braces, but I didn't get them until I was twelve. Can't we just wait until he's older?"

"Well," I replied, "I know John is a little young, but our best bet may be to do what we call Phase One treatment, which will likely include a limited number of braces and an expander … none of which will hurt," I quickly assured John.

"Cool!" said John. "When can we start?"

THE THREE QUESTIONS WE ASK
BEFORE RECOMMENDING BRACES

Before we recommend braces on children and adolescents, there are two overarching questions we ask:

- Will we miss a window of opportunity if we don't address this issue now?

- Will treatment now produce more stable results than if we waited to do braces at a later age?

- Can we achieve the same or a better result by holding off until more adult teeth are present?

Regardless of whether dentists refer patients to us for a specific reason, or they simply come in for a regular exam, the first thing we do is sit down and talk about any concerns. Then, during a child's initial exam, we'll look to see that all the teeth are where they're supposed to be. It's rather common for kids to have missing teeth or even extra teeth at this stage, so we do a general assessment, counting the teeth and looking at the relationship of the jaw to the teeth to see if there are any jaw discrepancies.

After that we'll often do a screening x-ray, or a whole-jaw film called a Panorex, just to make sure everything looks okay underneath the gums. Everything may look good on the surface, but you're only seeing a third of the tooth when you're looking in someone's mouth. An x-ray or Panorex will let us know if a tooth is developing in the wrong direction; how the adult teeth, which may not have erupted, are growing; and even if there are any issues with the roots that we couldn't detect during a visual exam.

Some parents are understandably hesitant to do this imaging, but thanks to today's technology, the amount of radiation is minimal. And without it, we really can't get a full picture of what's going on in your child's mouth.

Once we have all this information, we can make a recommendation as to what needs to be done. Oftentimes, it's nothing—the mouth could be developing beautifully, or the child could have a condition that we just want to keep under observation until he or she is a little older. Other times, we may need to do something right away so that we can take advantage of the window of opportunity.

WHEN IS EARLY TREATMENT BEST?

With younger, pre-adolescent children, the concern is usually jaw issues, such as overbites, underbites, crossbites, or excessive crowding that's not allowing room for the developing adult teeth. As recently as the 1980s and '90s, the most common answer to tooth crowding was to remove four adult teeth—usually one adult premolar tooth from each corner of the mouth. However, with this new dual-phase approach, we can take preventative steps to create room for tooth growth and often eliminate the need for extraction.

The greatest benefit to taking these preventative measures at younger ages, such as age seven, eight, or nine, is that younger jaws are much easier to influence. They still have a lot of growth ahead of them. Imagine how much more growth that John, at eight years old, has ahead of him versus a twelve-, thirteen-, or fourteen-year-old. At John's age, we can act now instead of allowing an unfavorable growth pattern to continue.

During phase one, treatment is directed at fixing these jaw issues, making room for the developing teeth to grow in, and reducing the severity of an existing condition. When we correct these jaw issues in phase one, we are giving our patients the biggest chance for success as the rest of their teeth develop. While some kids do not need phase two treatment, we find that most will still require further treatment in adolescence. Since correcting the *jaw* doesn't necessarily mean that the *teeth* are going to grow in straight or in the right position, we'll introduce full braces to address the teeth at around age twelve or so.

The most common conditions that we typically address with appliances or partial braces are:

• Crossbites

When the upper teeth are on the inside of the lower teeth. The most common crossbites are posterior (back teeth), however, we do see anterior (front teeth), crossbites as well. Treatment usually involves a palatal expander and mini-braces, which are placed on the adult teeth as well as on the specific baby teeth necessary for the correct movement.

- ## Underbites

When the lower jaw is too far forward in relation to the upper jaw. Treatment involves a combination of appliances and braces to move the upper jaw forward and the lower jaw, back.

- ## Severe Overbites (Overjets)

When the lower jaw is too far back in relation to the upper jaw. Treatment involves a combination of appliances and braces to move the upper jaw back, or restrain its growth, and to guide the lower jaw forward.

- ## Severe Crowding

When the adult teeth in the mouth are overlapping and the teeth are not yet erupted, or do not have sufficient room in the mouth to grow. Treatment involves a combination of expansion appliances to make more room, braces to move existing teeth into the most ideal position, and potentially the selective removal of baby teeth.

WHEN IS TREATMENT UNNECESSARY?

I'll be the first to say that orthodontists are totally biased. We can look into anyone's mouth and find something out of alignment, where maybe they just need a little space here or a rotation there. While we do want everyone to have a perfect smile, the reality is that not everyone requires orthodontics.

The two main reasons for undergoing orthodontic treatment are:

1. function

2.   aesthetics

People with poor function usually do not have good aesthetics, and people with good aesthetics only sometimes have proper poor function.

Orthodontics for Function

First, let's address function. Say you have one of the conditions listed earlier, such as a crossbite or crowding. These bad bites (what we call "malocclusions") put you at risk for:

- Excessive wear of your teeth

- Inability to chew properly

- Adverse speech effects

- Risk of jaw and joint issues

- Inability to properly clean your teeth, which puts you at risk for cavities and gum disease

If you have a "bad bite", then your dentist and your orthodontist will recommend treatment to improve your oral health conditions, your bite, and your smile.

Orthodontics for Aesthetics

Now let's say you have aesthetics concerns, such as spacing, minor crowding, or misalignment. While these do not affect your function or dental health, they certainly can influence your self-confidence. Whether we like it or not, we live in a culture that values appearance, regardless of age, and being able to take a good selfie is a high priority. If there's anything that's going to make you look and feel better about yourself, it's a straight, bright smile. However, if you don't mind not-so-perfect teeth, and the slight misalignment doesn't impact your mouth's ability to function, then orthodontics may not be necessary.

Is Invisalign an Option for Children?

Not yet. But stay tuned for this because with technological advances, this may very well become an option. When children have both adult and baby teeth—what's known as "mixed dentition"—those baby teeth are doing what they're supposed to do, which is maintaining function and space for the adult teeth and then falling out to allow the adult teeth to erupt. While this is happening, Invisalign can't do what it needs to do, which is grab onto the teeth and influence them in the appropriate direction. If a young patient's teeth are constantly falling out, for instance, then the aligners aren't going to fit well. The same goes for emerging adult teeth, which will push into the aligner as they grow in. Therefore, it's best to wait until you have all your adult teeth to do Invisalign.

NOT EVERYONE NEEDS BRACES

Braces aren't always just about functionality. Some people want them just so they can have that ideal smile. We'll let you know if you don't need them for functional purposes, such as correcting any of the jaw conditions we addressed earlier, but we'll be happy to talk about how braces can make an aesthetic difference. And if you're young and your bite is still developing, we'll keep an eye on them and make sure everything is developing properly. Ultimately, it's about how perfect you want your teeth to look and how ideal you want your bite to be. Sometimes a few months of braces can make a huge difference.

Not Your Parents' Braces

Technology for braces is getting better all the time. The experience is very different than it was in the 1980s or '90s. We're able to do things as of this writing (2018) that we couldn't even do *five* years ago, and the result is a much more comfortable experience with a much wider range of options.

The philosophy behind orthodontics has really experienced a paradigm shift in recent years. Practitioners have found that light, gentle forces create optimal tooth movement, which makes going through orthodontics more comfortable than ever before. I still remember my training at NYU when the senior member of the faculty would tell me, "You know you tightened their braces enough when you see tears in their eyes." Thankful, those days are long behind us.

Practitioners have found that light, gentle forces create optimal tooth movement, which makes going through orthodontics more comfortable than ever before.

Not only is the technology behind braces vastly improved, the experience as a patient does little to resemble what our generation (the parents) went through while having braces. Our offices are much more geared to a team approach, with staff playing a critical role in the process of aligning your teeth. Our highly trained team members have become true specialists within our office. While our treatment coordinators focus on helping you get started, some within our clinical staff may primarily deal with our youngest patients, while others may focus more on adults and Invisalign. Having specialists within the office vastly improves the quality of your experience and the level of service you are getting.

Ultimately, the best braces experiences are a direct result of how much responsibility you take in the process.

YOUR RESPONSIBILITIES WITH BRACES

Whether you're a child, adolescent, or adult, your responsibilities with braces are the same:

- **Take care of them!**

This means avoiding foods that could damage or break your braces, and it also means being careful not to pick at them or get involved in any activities that could damage them. If you need to wear rubber bands, wear them as often as they're prescribed.

Foods to Avoid While Wearing Braces

As a rule, you want to avoid foods that are too hard, sticky, or chewy. These include (but are not limited to):

Gum	Sticky and hard candy
Nuts	Ice
Corn chips	Pretzels
Sticky or hard chocolate	Hard cookies or crackers
Hard taco shells	Popcorn

Cut into smaller pieces, or avoid, the following:

Hard rolls	Fruit
Thin-crust pizza	Meat
Raw vegetables	Sub sandwiches
Croutons	Corn on the cob
French/Italian bread	Burgers

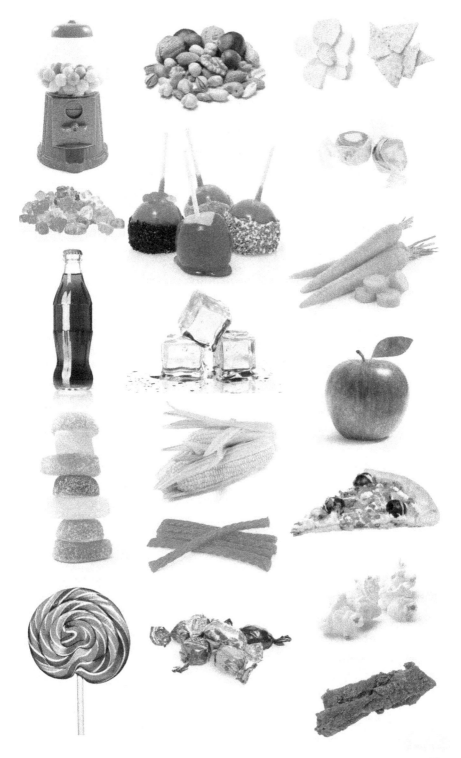

• Keep your appointments

The length of your appointments will vary depending on what we're trying to accomplish. For instance, there are times when we may not see you for ten weeks, and others when we ask you to come in every other week. This is because some treatments need more frequent check-ins than others. As a patient, keeping those appointments is one of the most important things you can do to get the best results.

These check-ins allow your orthodontist to adjust, repair, or make any other modifications necessary to bring your teeth into their ideal position and to keep your treatment moving along at a brisk pace. We've had some patients vanish for months on end and then wonder why their treatment is taking so long. The more proactive you are about your braces and care, the sooner you'll complete treatment.

It's also critical to keep appointments with your general or pediatric dentist while you're in orthodontic treatment. There is a common misconception that we, as orthodontists, are checking your teeth for cavities and cleaning them during visits. While we do polish your teeth when we're putting your braces on, this is only done to make sure the braces are firmly attached and does not constitute a true cleaning. And since our focus is on the alignment of your teeth and how they fit together, it's easy for a cavity or gum issue to go unnoticed. Our diagnostic imaging and standard practices also differ from those of a general dentist, all of which means that if we notice a cavity with the naked eye, it may have already progressed significantly.

Your general dentist, or your child's pediatric dentist, will need to monitor dental health during treatment to ensure that teeth are clean and to help catch any issues early on.

Your general dentist, or your child's pediatric dentist, will need to monitor dental health during treatment to ensure that teeth are clean and to help catch any issues early on. Braces can be a plaque and food trap, so more frequent cleanings may be necessary. In fact, we usually recommend scheduling a third cleaning with your dentist (most people have their teeth cleaned and examined twice a year) for the first year you are in braces, or undergoing orthodontic treatment, to give them an additional opportunity to monitor your progress and dental health during that time.

- ## Keep your teeth and braces clean

Healthy, clean teeth are always going to move faster and better than unhealthy ones. Inflamed gums are going to be resistant to movement and at the least will make that movement more uncomfortable. Poor gum health also increases the risk of demineralization (those white spots on your teeth) and cavities.

How Parents Can Help

It is not uncommon for us to see our patients for fifteen-minute appointments every six weeks. And as much as we try to reinforce the importance of this aspect of their treatment, we're also realistic about how much of what we say is retained by our younger patients, who may be texting away while in our chairs. Therefore, we often rely on parents to be our cheerleaders and coaches, encouraging their children to be responsible for the success of their treatment.

As a parent, your job (one of the many you may not have signed up for—sorry!) is to encourage your child to keep up with these three important responsibilities. If they do break a bracket or if something else goes wrong, call our office and we can give you instructions on the best way to handle it. Fortunately, not every broken bracket is an emergency that warrants running right in, but it's good to get them checked in a timely manner, since certain braces serve specific functions.

NO ONE EXCEPT YOUR ORTHODONTIST SHOULD DO YOUR BRACES

When I need a haircut, I know that I could just go to the local barber shop for a trim, but I choose to go to one of the more high-end salons. Why? Because they have some of the best stylists in town and their reputation reflects that. I see the value in their service and, if I do say so myself, I have never looked more handsome. The one thing I do *not* enjoy when I go there, however, are the other services that they push. They have a tooth-whitening kit that they offer me (they don't yet know that I'm a dentist), a woman who shows up once a week to provide Botox injections, and a part-time esthetician to do facials. While I may opt for the facial, I know that I will get much better tooth-whitening results from a cosmetic dentist, and if I want Botox, I'll be much better served by a plastic surgeon who has a far more intimate knowledge of the facial muscles and their interconnections, rather than having a floating person at my salon conduct the procedure.

Like anything else in life, you always want the best results. Therefore, you go to see the best people, because we all know that results can vary greatly. It's always better to see someone who lives and breathes a specific specialty rather than just a "dabbler." It doesn't matter what that specialty it is—people who just dabble in that procedure are not going to have the same level of training, nor will they have the same level of experience, as a specialist. Additionally, they won't know how to effectively deal with any problems that arise, as a specialist would.

For example, we have patients who come to us to have braces put on *because* they'd previously had braces put on by a dentist. Dentists do many things well, but just as you wouldn't see your general practitioner for a lung transplant, you shouldn't have a dentist performing a procedure that orthodontists do all day. Braces aren't just about straightening teeth—they're part of an intricate treatment that requires evaluation not only of the teeth but of the jaws and how the two relate to each other on complex levels.

Moving your teeth is not a commodity. It's not like buying contact lenses or glasses, where you see a specialist once and then fill a prescription wherever you like. Braces and the movement of teeth and jaws are a fine balance of art and science, and the training and skill of the person overseeing your case make a significant difference in the results you achieve.

We once had a dental hygienist come in as a patient for the reason mentioned above. The doctor she worked for did Invisalign for her after he attended a continuing-education training seminar, and she wore them for two and a half years. When she came to see us, her back teeth weren't even touching. Her bite was so bad in the back that we had to recalibrate a lot of factors to get her teeth back into a normal, functioning place. Then, because the total length of her treatment was so long, she ended having gum issues, as well, and had to see a periodontist to fix a problem that was much less likely to have occurred if she'd seen an orthodontist in the first place.

"CAN I JUST DO THE TOP?"

A common question that kids ask when getting braces is "Can I just do the top?" or "Can I just do the bottom?" With rare exceptions, the answer is "no." When you treat just one arch, it's hard to coordinate the teeth because you're unable to adjust the corresponding teeth either above or below. We need that coordination between top and bottom to get a good result. It is always a balance between esthetics and function. We not only want your teeth to look good, but to also function in a harmonious way with your opposing teeth, and when we treat only one arch it becomes very difficult to do that predictably.

Best Type of Braces for Younger Kids

Even though there are plenty of options out there for braces, including clear and lingual (braces that are placed on the tongue-side surface of teeth), young kids tend to do better with metal braces. This is because clear braces are made from a ceramic that's a little more fragile than metal, and with the rough and tumble life of most pre-adolescents, the sturdier their braces can be, the better. Metal braces also make it easier to do certain movements of the teeth that are a little more difficult to achieve with clear or lingual braces. Finally, there's the fun factor—with metal braces, kids get to pick out the colors of the elastic tie that holds the archwire in place against each bracket, and there are dozens of colors to choose from.

CHAPTER 5

It's Never Too Late to Go Straight

By Seth Newman, DDS

"All you orthodontists just sit around waiting for school to get out."

This was one of Dr. Jones's favorite jokes. He commonly said this during our many calls to discuss mutual patients. While that may have been the case at one time, it is certainly not the reality today. One-third of our patients are now adults, and that percentage continues to rise. And with that rise, a much greater proportion of our patients are being seen during the early part of the day.

When we look a little closer at our growing adult population, we also see that it's comprised of two-thirds adult females and one-third adult males. Many of these patients are in their twenties and thirties, but it's not uncommon to see adults in their sixties, seventies, and even eighties.

What's interesting to me is that at least half of our adult patients had braces as children or adolescents. Once again—as we like to say in orthodontics—"shift happens!"

As we like to say in ortho-dontics—"shift happens!"

Now, you may be thinking, "If half of adult patients had braces as a kid, then why get them at all? Why not wait to get braces as an adult?"

This is a great question and one that we do our best to answer, even though the explanation is not all that simple. As we discussed in earlier chapters, the main reason to have orthodontics as a child it to take advantage of that stage of rapid growth. The jaws and dentition of growing kids give orthodontists enormous advantages that we just don't have with the adult population. For instance, picture yourself at age thirteen. As good looking as you were back then, and despite how gracefully you've aged, not a lot about your appearance has remained constant. Your teeth really are no different. They exist in a dynamic body that is constantly undergoing changes and remodeling, which means that movement over time is normal and expected.

I've been impressed time and again by the dental IQ exhibited by adults who had braces as kids. They are often aware of what their teeth looked like when they originally finished orthodontics and how their teeth have shifted over the years. Since they already had perfect teeth, they want to preserve, or recreate, that and choose to address issues that others may consider minor.

On the other hand, adult patients who have not undergone orthodontics before usually decide to get them now for one of four reasons:

1. They always wanted straight teeth and a beautiful smile but couldn't afford it previously or could never find the right time to undergo treatment.

2. They're aware of the benefits of having straight teeth, including both the cosmetic and health benefits.

3. The treatment is being done in coordination with other dental work so that they have a strong foundation on which the additional dental procedures can be performed.

4. They are doing it for their significant others or are being encouraged by them to pursue orthodontics. We call these "the romantics."

NO AGE LIMIT TO BRACES

Not long ago we saw a woman named Brianna about her crowded lower teeth. After a quick exam, I assured her that we could not only straighten them, but that it wouldn't take too long to correct.

"If you don't mind me asking," I said after her consultation, "how old are you?"

"I don't mind at all," she said. "I'm eighty-eight."

"Why do you want to do this now?" I asked.

"Well, this one tooth has always bothered me, and I finally decided it was time to do something about it," she replied.

A set of lower braces and four months later we had her teeth straight, and she was happy as she could be.

There's really no age limit to when teeth can be straightened. More and more we're seeing older adults come in for consults and opting for either Invisalign or braces, because a straight smile is something they value for both aesthetic and health reasons. Straight teeth are much easier to keep clean, and a healthy mouth means a healthier body overall.

We all want to look good. The days of "I'm too old for braces" are over. Our mature patients are just as proud as our younger ones to have their teeth straighten. In fact, it's not uncommon for moms to go through treatment at the same time as their kids, often electing to do Invisalign while their child is in braces. In one memorable case, we had a seventy-three-year-old grandmother undergo orthodontics at the same time as her granddaughter. The best part was that they both chose to get metal braces so that they could look like twins.

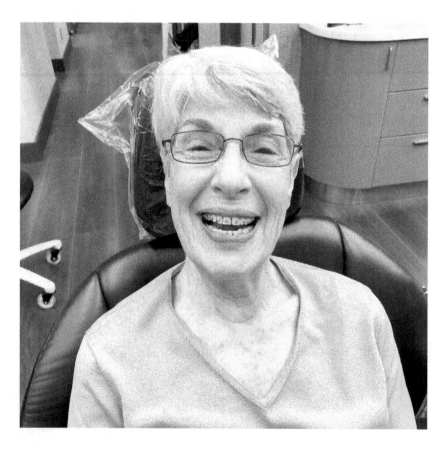

When treating adult patients, there's usually a higher level of coordination needed between the dentist and orthodontist. Most importantly, we want to make sure their gums and bone levels are healthy enough to undergo orthodontics. This is rarely a problem, though, especially for those patients who see their dentist regularly for checkups and cleanings.

One concern that we do keep top of mind is how orthodontics is going to affect any pre-existing crowns or bridges, which were built to the patient's original bite (or occlusion). While it's our goal to put all their teeth in the most ideal and harmonious position, these pre-existing conditions often warrant a discussion with the patient's dentist to determine if any of the existing dental work needs to be replaced. Sometimes, especially if a restoration has been in place for a while, we're able to coordinate an ideal time to have those elements replaced after orthodontics.

HEY MOM AND DAD, YOU DESERVE A GREAT SMILE, TOO

Eric came in with his twelve-year-old daughter, Marlowe, for her first six-week checkup after getting braces, and for the first time, casually said something to me about his teeth.

We'd seen Eric off-and-on since Marlowe was seven years old. She came in not long after her birthday, which wasn't a surprise since her mom was a local dentist and knew the importance of seeing an orthodontist at that age. Plus, she'd noticed that Marlowe's teeth looked a little crowded and she wanted us to take a look.

Marlowe's mom was right, and fortunately, we caught it at the best possible time. Starting with Phase One treatment while she still had her baby teeth, we got her jaws in just the right place and, with a few minor exceptions, Eric was there with her for every appointment.

I'd noticed that Eric's teeth looked a little crowded from a distance, but it wasn't until he asked me what I thought of them that I realized the severity of it. The treatment would be pretty involved, I explained, and could take up to a year and a half to complete.

"Ah, I'm not doing that," he said, brushing it off. His wife, he explained, had been on him for some time to get them straightened out, but he just didn't want to deal with it.

As we continued to see Marlowe for her six-week checkups, however, Eric began to ask more and more questions about the various potential procedures that would apply to him, and I could tell he was warming up to the idea. Then, on Marlowe's fifth follow-up, he decided he was ready to go for it.

Eric opted for clear braces instead of Invisalign because in his own words, "I want you guys to do all the work." Instead of remembering to switch out trays every week or so, all he needed to do was keep his regular appointments. Once he got started, it was surprising how motivated he was to complete his treatment. He came in every three weeks for checkups and completed his case in nine months, which is well ahead of what I originally told him and less than the twelve- to eighteen-month average for most of our adult patients.

CHOOSING THE RIGHT APPLIANCE

We try to give our patients what they want, as long as it's feasible. While we can accommodate their wishes most of the time, it's also our job as doctors to prevent our patients from making the wrong choices. "Non-malfeasance" is one of the most important tenets of the clinical practice.

Angela was a vibrant twenty-one-year-old junior in college with teeth that looked straight enough that her parents hadn't thought she needed orthodontics. It wasn't until she had her wisdom teeth taken out that a panoramic x-ray revealed that she had an impacted canine. It turned out that a baby canine was still in place in her upper jaw. Up until that moment, Angela had just thought she had one particularly small tooth that was narrower and shorter than the rest.

During her initial consultation, one of the first statements she made was, "There's no way I'm getting braces."

"I completely understand where you're coming from," I said, so we spent a while talking about why the idea of braces was such a negative for her. It turned out that what she really objected to was having braces during the business-school interviews she would be going through during her senior year. She already felt as though she appeared young, and braces, she thought, would only make her look younger.

Since Invisalign wasn't an option in this case (there's just not a predictable way to use the Invisalign process to bring in an impacted canine) we talked about-fixed appliance options. Then I introduced her to Taylor, our scheduling coordinator, who was wearing clear braces with tooth-colored wires. Angela was stunned because she hadn't even noticed them when Taylor greeted her. That, and the fact that the process could be done in a year or less (Angela had been convinced it would take two or three years), was encouraging enough for her to agree to wear ceramic braces. She ended up with amazing results—and best of all, the braces were off by the time grad school interviews came around.

Some appliances are more suited for certain treatments, but if someone comes in with an appliance in mind, we're going to try to make it work. For patients with a severe overbite, for instance, we often recommend Invisalign, because with braces, they run the risk of biting onto the brackets. Other times we may suggest combined treatment modalities so that patients get what they want, while we still achieve a successful outcome. If someone has a severely rotated tooth in the back, for instance, we may suggest sectional braces (that is, just a few braces) to get the tooth turned around just enough so that we can complete the case with Invisalign.

It's our job to educate our patients and explain why something may or may not be a good idea. Ideally, we end up aligning our patients' needs with the technical aspects of their case. Our patients expect a beautiful smile and it's our job to deliver the proper balance of aesthetics and function. Perhaps most importantly of all, we ensure that we can align the expectations, needs, and desires of our patients with the abilities (and in some cases, limitations) of the various treatment modalities and appliances. Aligning expectations with attainability is significant in many facets of our lives, and orthodontic treatment is no exception.

Clear Braces vs. Invisalign

The clear braces we have today are amazing. Since they're made with zirconium, they're incredibly clear, and the wires are made of ionized metal that makes them hard to see unless you know what you're looking for.

I had an opportunity to wear clear braces for several months and was surprised at how few people noticed them. This helped me realize that something that may seem like a big, glaring change for us is practically unnoticeable to others.

One of the benefits of braces over Invisalign, as Eric found out earlier in this chapter, is the low involvement on the part of the patient. We do all the work for you. As a patient, all you need to do is show up for your appointments and maintain good oral hygiene, which includes taking good care of your braces. There are no trays to switch out or possibly lose, and you can't forget to put them on at night or in the morning. One good way to determine if braces are better for you than Invisalign is to ask yourself if you tend to forget minor tasks, such as watering the plants. If so, then braces might be the way to go.

On the other hand, if you don't keep clear braces incredibly clean, it's going to show. Braces tend to trap food, which means you're going to have to spend more time keeping both your braces and your teeth clean. And even though a lot of people may not notice you're wearing braces, Invisalign is still going to provide better visual aesthetics than braces.

As for Invisalign, being able to take the trays (also called "aligners") out can be a huge benefit. You have the option of taking them off for special occasions, like for a night out, or if you're giving a big presentation at work. There are also no food restrictions as there are with braces, and your dental-hygiene regime is no different than when you were undergoing orthodontics. Additionally, they're much less noticeable than clear braces, and even on close inspection, can be hard to spot.

Lingual Braces

As the name implies, lingual braces are placed on the tongue-side of the teeth. Since no part of the braces is on the outside of the teeth, lingual braces are the only option that is completely invisible. This makes them even more aesthetically pleasing than clear ceramic braces or Invisalign. They really are an excellent orthodontic option for patients who want all the benefits of braces without the chance that they'll be noticed.

Just as with patients in ceramic braces, we usually recommend that our adult patients in lingual braces come in every three weeks over the course of treatment, which usually takes about a year to complete. It's an excellent option for those patients who want maximum aesthetics and do not want to worry about the compliance concerns that come with wearing clear aligners.

The downside, however, is that the cost of lingual braces is significantly higher than our other orthodontic options due to the cost of the appliances themselves, as well as the technical aspects of treatment with lingual braces. It typically takes considerably more doctor time than is necessary with other appliances. Additionally, some patients may experience tongue and speech issues after initial placement, although these challenges are usually short lived.

We typically use lingual braces either on patients who don't want to wear clear aligners, or because the case was too technically challenging for Invisalign. Since Invisalign's effectiveness has improved so much in recent years, however, we've found ourselves recommending lingual braces with less and less frequency.

PARTNERING UP FOR A BRILLIANT SMILE

It is not uncommon for us to encounter patients with missing teeth. Sometimes these are children or young adults who were born with missing teeth (what we call "congenitally missing teeth" and which usually involve the upper lateral teeth, or one or more of the premolar teeth), but more often they occur in adult patients who have lost their teeth due to dental breakdown, root canals, extractions, or any number of reasons.

Treating mouths with missing teeth are some of our most rewarding cases, as we get to conduct treatment in conjunction with our dental colleagues. These multi-specialty interdisciplinary cases are usually done so that the orthodontist can place the existing teeth in the most ideal position to allow the next doctor to work his or her magic. This may be a general dentist or any number of dental specialists, including prosthodontists, oral surgeons, periodontists, endodontists, implantologists, or restorative dentists. We often tell our patients that these co-treatment cases are like building a house, with orthodontics handling the foundation. When you have a solid foundation, anything you build on it is going to be that much sounder.

Another condition we commonly encounter is that of small or chipped front teeth. For these cases, we work

When you have a solid foundation, anything you build on it is going to be that much sounder.

with restorative dentists to prepare the teeth for more cosmetic procedures, such as bonding or veneers. These cases require careful coordination among specialties. Sometimes a millimeter of space here or there can make all the difference in how well the restorative dentist can create an ideal smile. For this reason, we'll often have the other dentist approve all the spacing prior to removing braces, and it's also why there may be many visits with various doctors before a patient is deemed ready to move on to the next step.

One of the more exciting procedures we do for those patients requiring implants is called "implant site development." If a patient has been missing a tooth for a certain number of years, it's not uncommon for the bone at the site of the missing tooth to degrade. Since a tooth root is no longer occupying this highly specialized bone, the bone is no longer receiving the message to stick around, so it gets slowly reabsorbed over time, rendering that part of the jaw less able to support the surgical placement of an implant.

In these cases, we rebuild the site so that an implant can assume the location of the missing tooth root. To do this, we'll gradually move a tooth into that area, let the bone build back up around it, and then gradually move it back out again. The bone that built up will remain for some time before the body is triggered to reabsorb it, so once the site is ready we send the patient on to the restorative dentist or surgeon to have the implant placed.

Without the help of an orthodontist, placing an implant where a tooth has been missing for some time—or where a tooth failed to grow in at all—would be an impossible task. Alternatively, it would involve more than one surgical procedure to artificially build the bone up or to graft it. These are invasive and costly procedures and only give the benefit to that single site, ignoring all other possible areas that can be improved.

SPEEDING UP THE STRAIGHTENING PROCESS

It truly is an exciting time to be going through orthodontics, and one of the newest technological innovations is that of *accelerated tooth movement.*

Life happens quickly—and now, so can your teeth. You may suddenly find yourself engaged to be married in six months, or if you're an international student, you may have only a short time in the States and want to have dental work done while you're here. No matter the reason, sometimes you need to have your teeth moved, and you need to do it quickly. In these cases, there are ways to accelerate your treatment using different devices and procedures.

AcceleDent is probably our most popular accelerated-orthodontic procedure. This hands-free device is designed to encourage faster tooth movement and is used in conjunction with braces or aligners to rapidly straighten teeth. AcceleDent uses SoftPulse Technology to help your current treatment work faster by generating small vibrations called micro-pulses to gently accelerate the movement of your teeth as they are guided by the orthodontics. These micro-pulses speed up the remodeling process of the bones in the mouth, thus accelerating tooth movement.

Patients who use the device find it very comfortable to wear; all they need to do is to find a continuous twenty-minute window to wear it. The hardest part of the treatment is that you can't talk while wearing it, so many patients use it while commuting in the car or while watching a show.

AcceleDent claims that it can help patients move their teeth up to 40 percent faster than traditional orthodontic movements. While I can't confirm that the procedure cuts treatment time by as much as the company claims, I have seen meaningful accelerated movement of teeth with regular use.

Propel is another device we use for a procedure called micro-osteoperforation. This device creates a series of small alveolar micro-osteoperforations in the gums, which are little holes in the gum and bones. This stimulates the surrounding bone and works with the patient's own biology to accelerate tooth movement. This is an excellent technology for site-specific areas where we want to encourage rapid tooth movement. The healing process in a local area recruits cells that are involved in bone turnover and uses a biological "hack" to trick the body into getting things moving faster.

THE SURGICAL OPTION

In some cases, braces aren't enough to straighten teeth or bring them close to an ideal bite. If the root cause of a malocclusion (bad bite) is jaw-related instead of tooth-related, then there is a limit to what we can correct with orthodontics alone. Major skeletal discrepancies such as a large overbite, underbite, or open bite in fully grown adults may need orthognathic (jaw) surgery to correct the jaw discrepancy and bring the teeth into alignment.

With a patient who may require orthognathic surgery in conjunction with orthodontics, the first step is to create a comprehensive set of records. We then insist that these patients see a surgeon prior to beginning orthodontics, so that they can fully understand what is involved in their treatment. We often say that the orthodontics is the easier part of their treatment; therefore, we want our patients to be fully committed to the surgery before we begin.

For these procedures, patients usually wear braces for anywhere from six months to a year before the surgery to bring the teeth into the most ideal position. The orthognathic surgeon then uses the teeth as a guide to reset the jaws into the right place, aligning the teeth and then fastening the jaws in the correct position. After surgery, patients will typically spend an additional three to six months in braces as their jaws heal and their teeth settle into the new positions.

The results we can achieve for these patients are dramatic. Careful coordination is needed between the orthodontist and oral surgeon, but these are some of the most rewarding cases for us. As mentioned earlier, there is great reward in restoring someone's function and aesthetics in concert with our colleagues in an interdisciplinary manner.

We are not only changing smiles but also faces, and these are some of those rare opportunities to truly improve someone's life through treatment.

CHAPTER 6

When Am I Done, Will It Hurt & How Much Will It Cost?

By Efstathios Giannoutsos, DDS

"When am I done?" "Will it hurt?" "How much will it cost?" These are the three most universal questions asked at our offices.

"WHEN AM I DONE?"

This is the question we are asked more than any other over the course of the day. There are days when we joke that it's like being on a road trip where the kids are constantly asking, "Are we there yet?"—except you can't just say, "We'll be there when I say so." All joking aside, as much as we hear this question, we respect that it is very important to the person asking and we do our best to give an honest and sincere answer.

This question is often asked when patients are feeling a little duress about their procedures. They may have begun treatment with all the excitement in the world. Some of them want to truly correct their teeth, others want them because their friends have them—but once they have the appliances on, and the novelty wears off, without fail, their focus begins to shift to when they can have the braces off.

When we do answer this question, it's very important that we give patients our best educated guess, so that they don't become discouraged—even if it's not the answer they were hoping to hear. Orthodontics is very dependent on patient cooperation. Everything from keeping your teeth clean to regularly wearing elastics to not breaking braces and wires can have a real impact on the outcomes we achieve and the time it takes to complete treatment. For this reason, when we answer this question we also try to explain what we're aiming to achieve, to help the patient facilitate the outcome.

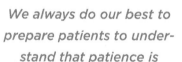

We always do our best to prepare patients to understand that patience is needed in orthodontics.

Prior to beginning treatment, we always do our best to prepare patients to understand that patience is needed in orthodontics. We find that when we can provide information about the physiology of tooth movement (teeth are actually moving through bone) the more aligned their expectations become with the timing of treatment. As much as we would like to believe we are getting our message across, we all have selective memories, especially with children and adolescents who don't tend to think about what life will be like day-to-day with braces. Ultimately, we just have to wait and let them come to us with the inevitable question.

Answering that question, however, isn't as simple as counting days and pointing to a specific calendar date. First, we must identify what "done" is.

With one of my patients, whom we'll call Janet, the first thing we did after her consultation and imaging (x-rays, models, and pictures) was to pull up a stock image of what an ideal bite looks like—perfect alignment between the jaws with no spacing or crowding—and place it side by side with an image of her own deep overbite.

"If this," I said, pointing to the stock image, "is a perfect, one hundred percent score, then the position of your teeth right now is at about thirty percent. It's our goal to get your teeth to as close to one hundred percent as possible. Of course, no mouth is ever actually one hundred percent, but it's the ideal we shoot for."

In her case, we not only needed to correct her overbite, we also had to space out and straighten her crowded bottom teeth and have her dentist build up her lateral incisors to a proper size. This was because they were small for her face and not in proportion to the neighboring teeth. If we could address all those problem areas, we could get her close to that 100 percent ideal—or at least into the lower 90 range, for sure. However, it wasn't going to be a quick process. Every bite has its own qualities and challenges, and while technology, patient education, and clinician savvy have all increased over the years, resulting in reduced treatment time, specific end dates are still hard to pin down.

Say a patient starts with Phase One treatment, which usually begins around eight or nine years of age, when patients have their upper and lower anterior (front) teeth and their first molars. Treatment length at this age is typically between nine and fifteen months, and we finish most of these cases in less than twelve months.

For someone who's dentally mature (has all the adult teeth in place, or whose teeth are on their way into the mouth), that same procedure may take eighteen to twenty-four months. However, that time may be less if the patient went through Phase One treatment, where a lot of the jaw-specific issues are handled early. It can also be longer and involve the need to extract teeth if we have not undergone this first phase of treatment.

For instance, we may spend twelve months on a treatment, tackle some major issues, and get the patient looking great, but the bite still might not be perfect. In that case, we might spend an additional six months really nailing down the bite and getting it as close to perfect as possible. The treatment may not be done on the date we were shooting for, but the result is a bite that's that much closer to ideal.

The way I explain it to our patients is to think of the orthodontic procedure in the same way you would think about having a house built. Say your contractor originally told you that he could build your house in six months, but his team encountered some unexpected challenges. Should he deliver a half-finished house to you, or would you rather have the project seen through to completion?

Challenges are rife in the orthodontic world. No two patients will react the same way to the same treatment, because no two craniofacial structures are the same. Think about the last time you walked up to a group of people: every single one of them had a different facial structure—different bite, different jaw set, and different colors, sizes, and shapes of teeth. It's these variations that make it so hard to pin down an exact date for treatment completion.

One of the most important things we can do when asked the question "When am I done?" is to educate and encourage the patient to comply with the procedure as much as possible to complete treatment as soon as possible. If our patients buy into and understand that we're not trying to "hold them hostage" by keeping them in treatment longer but are simply trying to give them the best possible smile, then the remaining treatment time will go a lot more smoothly.

When we begin treatment, we always give patients a range, from most optimistic completion date to most pessimistic. This is usually an educated guess we make based on our experiences with treating similar conditions. We are usually close to our range, mainly because we're great believers in the adage "under-promise and over-deliver." This means that if we think your treatment is going to take about twelve to fifteen months to complete, we'll probably tell you it's going to take fifteen to eighteen months, so that if it's shorter, you'll be pleasantly surprised; and if it takes a little longer, we've given ourselves a little bit of a cushion.

Often, it's not until we've completed the first third of a case that we get to see how patient is responding to treatment, whether he or she is complying with the treatment (and if so, how much), and how the teeth are moving. Oftentimes we surprise ourselves by how fast we're able to accomplish a treatment, and we finish prior to an original estimate.

THE IMPORTANCE OF INVOLVING THE DENTIST

As we near the end of treatment, we like to ask a patient's dentist what he or she thinks about the progress, just in case that professional can identify something specific about a patient's condition or growth pattern that we hadn't considered before. For instance, a patient may have a tooth with a history of being problematic or may have taken longer to recover from other procedures such as gum grafting or implants. All this information gives us a much clearer idea of what to expect in terms of progress and completion of treatment.

Additionally, and just as importantly, we need feedback while our appliances are still in place and our patients are still motivated. When dentists are clear with us up-front about how they would like to see their patients' bite and smile set up, then we're much better prepared to bring those patients to an ideal finish. Imagine if your dentist didn't get to look at your mouth at all until after your treatment was complete, then noticed that there were some issues that needed attention or refinement! It's much better for our patients when dentists are able to make such observations while treatment is taking place, so we can make those important changes.

So—when are you done? You're done when your teeth are perfect. You're done when you love your teeth, your general dentist loves your teeth, the people closest to you love your teeth, and your orthodontist loves your teeth. That is a lot of love going into your smile!

GRADUAL RESULTS IN AN INSTANT-GRATIFICATION WORLD

We're in an age of instantaneous everything, with information at our fingertips and the ability to get just about anything we want with a single click. Today, you can find a place to stay, a significant other to go with you, and a ride share to drive you there in less than four minutes. And you can make these arrangements on the bus or while walking, using only your smartphone! With that in mind, it makes sense that a lot of people have a tough time with how long it takes to move teeth and complete orthodontic treatment.

We always make it a point to emphasize the length of treatment time that an individual is going to need at the outset. But even then, we have a few patients who can't take the wait. We notice when they start to unravel at the seams, becoming more and more anxious about completing the treatment. When that happens, we do our best to remind them of the results we're shooting for and the progress we've made so far—but if they just can't take wearing their appliances any longer, then we'll compromise. It may be a negotiation regarding function or aesthetics, or the risk of a longer-term challenge, but we'll bring them to as stable a place as we can get at that point in their treatment and cut them loose.

A young woman named Karla was a great example of this. She was a beautiful girl, and she wanted her teeth to be perfect, but to get her to an aesthetic and functional ideal wasn't going to be a speedy process. We'd need at least a year, I told her, and explained exactly what we needed to do and how we needed to move her teeth.

She didn't love the idea that the treatment would take more than a few weeks, however.

"Look," I explained, "creating a beautiful smile that lasts a lifetime requires fundamental changes that take time. It's a big commitment to get there, but it's for the long-term health and wellness of your body."

"Yeah, yeah, I'm sure you'll be able to figure something out," she said.

This was a girl who was clearly not accustomed to hearing the word "no," and I couldn't find another way to explain that the process was going to take far longer than a few weeks. Still, she wanted to move forward, so I made sure to document our conversation via email, including her mother and father on it, so that everything was abundantly clear on the recommended procedure and how long it could possibly take.

Inevitably, three months into her treatment, Karla informed me that her braces had to come off and that her teeth weren't perfect. I simply showed her the email and said, "I understand what you want, but there's simply no way we can get your teeth where you want them to be in this length of time."

"Okay," she said, "then take them off."

I agreed, but before taking them off, I asked her to give me at least six to eight weeks to take care of some major concerns, such as spaces that needed to be closed and a problem with the way that two of her teeth came together in the back, She allowed me the time, and seven weeks later, I removed her braces and put her in permanent retainers so that the changes we made would at least be as stable as possible.

A little over one year later she came back in and asked to be fitted with Invisalign. She'd finally accepted how long it would take to achieve the results she wanted, but she had to make that decision to move forward on her own. Sometimes people need to make decisions on their own terms. That's okay with us—as long as we're communicating well and openly throughout.

"I'M DONE"

Even though we don't recommend it, there are times when we're asked to pause or stop treatment before it's done. Bar and bat mitzvahs, for instance, as well as confirmations, graduations, weddings, or other major life events that come up before treatment is complete may result either in the use of accelerated-orthodontics or just the acceptance that this is as good as we're going to get for now.

Sometimes patients want their braces removed for important events, such as a "Sweet Sixteen," and then replaced right after the event. Unfortunately, it isn't an easy thing to do; when braces are removed, even if it's for a short period of time, it can take up to several months to get everything back to where they were at the time the braces were removed. When we put on a new set of braces, we need to start with a very thin wire again until we can build back up to thicker, more rigid wires. However, if our patients understand the that we may lose some time by doing this, we're always going to do what we can to make them happy.

We always try to talk patients away from this decision, but ultimately, the choice is in their hands. We're not going to make anyone do anything they don't want to do. We're partners in this process, and when patients want to back out, we're not going to stop them.

"WILL IT HURT?"

The short answer is, yes, there is minor discomfort. That's the bad news. The good news is that we can minimize it and control it dramatically.

There are two types of discomfort that we encounter as part of orthodontic procedures. There's the irritation of having a new appliance in your mouth, rubbing against the cheeks, lips, and tongue until those areas grow accustomed to the change. This usually takes about two or three days at most. To ease this, we provide patients with a special combination of silicone and wax that they can apply to help relieve the areas being irritated.

Then there's the ache that results from activating the whole orthodontic system. Once the wire is attached to the braces it's like a sudden bear hug in the mouth, which isn't painful per se, but does feel a little tight and has often been called both uncomfortable and annoying by our patients. Patients describe the same feelings when their Invisalign aligners are in.

The next day is when the aching begins, which is similar to the discomfort you feel after a really good workout, especially if you haven't been to the gym in a while. This pain—counterintuitively—is actually a good thing, because it lets you know that progress is being made; teeth are moving and you're on your way to an ideal bite and smile. But because it can be uncomfortable at first, we typically prescribe acetaminophen, ibuprofen, or something similar, to be taken both before we put braces on (what we call "preemptive pain management") and then as needed afterward as needed for pain. We recommend doing this for the first two or three visits for two reasons:

1. the height of discomfort reaches a much lower peak

2. the length of time in that lower degree of discomfort is much shorter

Everyone's tolerance for discomfort is different. Most of our patients don't need to take anything. However, for those who feel they need it, we are sympathetic to their concern. We also teach them that they have control over this discomfort and that we can ensure they do not reach their personal "peak pain," whatever that might mean for each individual. At all times, we make sure that this decreased amount of discomfort lasts for the shortest time that is biologically possible.

Despite the discomfort inherent in these procedures, we've never had a patient who couldn't tolerate it. Children as young as seven up to elderly adults and even special-needs patients have all been able to take the treatment in stride. There have been times when our younger patients cry from the anticipation of getting braces, but once we start the procedure, they realize that the placement of the braces is not going to hurt, so they really begin to ease into the treatment and relax.

It can be incredibly rewarding to watch these patients as they transition from a place of fear and anxiety to being excited to sit in our chair over the course of only a few short visits. It's wonderful to see them realize how much stronger they are than they thought they were and understand that everything is going to be alright.

This was the case with a little boy named Mikey who came to us for braces. During his visit, he was so nervous that he had tears in his eyes and wouldn't let go of his mom's hand. But by the end of the treatment, he was so comfortable that he fell asleep in the chair. I had to wake him up at the end of the appointment to tell him we were done! Now that's what I would call a good day for me, and a great day for Mikey and his mom.

Once the braces are in place, we give each new patient a special Survival Kit. This includes everything you need to take care of your braces, toothbrushes, floss, wax, home care instructions and most importantly, a special gift (we like to keep that as a surprise). We also give detailed lessons in how to apply wax, smooth sharp edges, and clip wires if they need to. When it comes to braces, we give our patients carte blanche to do whatever they need to do to make themselves or their children comfortable. We remind them that there's no need to fret if something breaks—we'll be able to take care of it, and the kit includes pretty much everything you need to keep you comfortable until we can see you.

From the very first call to our offices, it's our goal to give our patients a five-star experience, and control over the process is a big part of that. Along with the Survival Kit, we offer printed material, instructional videos, access to us via our website and by phone, and people at our offices who can triage when needed. Most importantly, we remind our patients that this is not a paternal "do-it-or-else" kind of environment. We're partners in this process, and we're here for you.

"HOW MUCH WILL IT COST?"

There is a trifecta of requirements that must be met before we move forward with any procedure:

1. There must be a desire for treatment.

2. There must be a need and benefit for treatment.

3. The treatment must work for you as a patient and/or patient's parent.

When we have a recommended treatment and these conditions are met, then we can move forward to discuss costs, at which point we do everything we can to have complete transparency about our expenses and explaining what they mean.

There is not a week that goes by that we don't get a phone call from someone asking a variation of: "how much do braces cost?" Similarly, it's not uncommon for that to be one of the first questions we are asked during the initial consultation. While by no means do we want to minimize the fee, we have found through experience that this question is often asked when patients aren't sure what else to ask. Our goal is to build value to everything for our treatment. When we review with our new patients not only all aspects of their malocclusion but also what they can expect every step along the way of their treatment, they have a true understanding of our fees.

Cost Is Patient-Dependent

While it is true that most of our patients fall into a pre-determined fee range that is dependent on their treatment needs, there are multiple factors that come into play when quoting cost to patients, apart from what insurance covers, and most of those factors are patient-dependent. Our fees are ultimately customized for the specifics of each individual case to fit the needs and desires of our patients. We understand that orthodontics can be a large expense for families, and we do our best to balance that understanding with all that is needed to support quality orthodontic care.

The good news is that we do not believe in charging for an initial consultation. We made that decision long ago because we want our patients to meet us first. This gives us an opportunity to gain their trust and confidence, and to let them see our office and meet our staff before deciding to go with us for their orthodontic treatment. This consultation also gives us the opportunity to be totally transparent about our treatment philosophies and review the costs before we ever get started.

During this consultation, the first thing we need to determine is the type of treatment needed and the best way to approach it. Once we've identified the need, then we usually have our patients sit down with one of our treatment coordinators to review the tentatively proposed treatment plan, our fees, as well as their out-of-pocket and insurance-covered costs.

While the way in which we structure our fees and payment plans has not considerably changed, the benefits that our patients have is always evolving. It is not uncommon for patients and parents to assume that if they have insurance, the cost of treatment will be fully covered. Yet, while the ways in which patients qualify for ortho-dontics benefits has changed, the dollar amount which insurance companies cover has not. In the late 1980s, the average patient had a lifetime orthodontic benefit of $1,500, and this amount remains the same as of 2018. Clearly, orthodontic coverage is not dissimilar to other dental coverage, which means it is often limited in scope.

Over the years, there has really been no adjustment for inflation or fee increases, which means the amount of coverage people have is a lot less today than it used to be. And not only is the amount of coverage less, it is also harder to qualify. Age restrictions, as well some insurance companies covering only what they deem to be "handicapping malocclusions" makes it a lot harder to qualify for benefits. Also, this "once-in-a-lifetime maximum" is in stark contrast to regular dental coverage, which renews annually.

This means that most of the cost for treatment is an out of pocket expense and consequently, many of our patients choose one of our many flexible payment plans.

Financing Made Easy

We recently partnered with an amazing company—OrthoFi—for handing patient finances. This system not only keeps everything honest and transparent, but it also comes with the patient option of extending payment terms out for well over three years. If a patient has insurance, for instance, we use the OrthoFi system to determine that patient's benefit level and look to how we can maximize that as much as possible. OrthoFi advocates for our patients and ensures that there is electronic proof of their contract with their respective insurance companies, keeping those insurance companies on their toes and honest in ways that are impractical for our staff to keep up with consistently. Also, we now have recorded proof of the contact we have made with the insurance company on our patients' behalf.

One of the features that we are most excited about with OrthoFi is called the Payment Slider, which gives patients the freedom to choose the down payment that best fits them. If they want to start with as little as $250 down, not problem; just slide to the left, and the slider shows what the monthly payment will be. Want to save some money on the fee? Then slide all the way to the right, and take advantage of our payment-in-full discount. OrthoFi allows us to work with our patients to help them build payment plans that fit.

The ultimate question that our patients need to answer is, "What is the value that you, the individual or parent, assign to your best smile, the best bite that we can give you, which you'll have for the rest of your life?"

If you think about it, every day we assign value to things, whether it's what to spend on a new car, a new outfit, or a new pair of shoes. Most of those things are assets with inherent declining value. A new car drops in value the second you drive it off the lot. The new outfit is now used, and those shoes are worn—whereas the reverse is true for your smile. Starting with the increase in your own sense of self-worth, a healthy, straight smile has a direct impact on other people's first impression of you and how they interact with you. It has an incredibly positive relationship with you and a correlation to *your* opinion of yourself. By comparison, the time and money spent on orthodontics is small compared to the impact that a beautiful smile has over a lifetime.

CHAPTER 7

The Patient Experience

By Efstathios Giannoutsos, DDS

The patient experience does not start when you walk into our office lobby—it begins when you first hear about us. Maybe your dentist recommended us, or it could have been a friend. It's also possible that some of our online or off-line marketing caught your attention and attracted you to us. We take our reputation very seriously and believe that a referral is the highest compliment that we can receive. That is why we want to impress you with your first phone call—and why we do everything we can so that you love us every step of the way.

It's our goal from the very beginning to give you, the patient, the best experience possible and to make sure you understand that:

1. We appreciate you considering us for your, or your child's, treatment.

2.   We want to provide you with the best understanding possible of who we are, what we do in general, and what we can do for you specifically.

In everything we do, our goal is to provide an experience that is professional, friendly, and welcoming.[1] When patients call our office, we want them to feel like they are calling a friend or a cousin, so they'll know that they are an extended part of our orthodontic family. Whether you're calling to book the first appointment for you or your child, or you've been seeing us every three months for a year, calling our offices should be an easy conversation that leaves you feeling confident and informed.

FUNCTIONAL PROCESS, FUNCTIONAL SPACE

We pride ourselves on creating an office environment that reflects our desire to provide both functional and state-of-the-art services. Our spaces are heavily design-focused; highly functional and welcoming; and they have great flow, well-lit spaces, and very clean lines. This is especially important due to the nature of orthodontic offices; on any given day, our offices are functioning with the speed and choreography of a fine local restaurant. If you're a regular, our front desk staff will know your name, your kids' names, your preferences, and anything else necessary to give you the best possible experience.

On that first visit, we're cognizant of the fact that you're assessing our functionality and aesthetics. You're paying attention to who greets you, how we handle check-in, and how long the wait appears to be. And how we handle this part of the process will likely play a

---

1   We should also mention *fast!* See chapter 9 for information about the OrthoFi system—which allows patients to fill out all their paperwork in advance of the first appointment.

big role into whether you ditch us that day and never come back, or you become a part of our orthodontic family for years to come.

WHAT TO EXPECT FROM YOUR FIRST VISIT

Depending on whether this is your first visit or a return appointment, we'll send you in one of two directions when you come in. For your first visit, we'll get you into an empty chair or private room as quickly as possible, where you get to know our treatment coordinator. The coordinator will introduce him- or herself, tell you a little bit about our practice, who we are, what we do, when we're open, what we specialize in, and just run through a quick summary to help orient you.

Then, since we've already reviewed the medical history you submitted through OrthoFi before you arrived, the treatment coordinator will just ask some simple questions such as "Who is your regular dentist?" and "Is there anything else we need to know about your medical history?" Then we delve straight into why you're here and what your chief concern is.

Once the treatment coordinator is done with the introductions, he or she will bring the doctor into the mix. If there were any dental films sent through email by your dentist or by you or through OrthoFi, the doctor will have reviewed those, along with your medical records, to be well informed before walking in.

Then the exploration and assessment phase begins. One of the first things we like to do when we meet a new patient is ask a few pertinent questions and then sit back and listen. In our experience, both as a patient and in observing other practitioners, too many doctors of every specialty talk *at* you as opposed to speaking *with* you

They are quick to focus in on the issue at hand. In orthodontics, it's usually some misaligned teeth. Then they go straight into how they are going to fix the problem.

We are strong believers that a clinician can miss some critical insight into patients' motivations and what is truly important to them with this approach. In spending some extra time, we get to know our patients as people, and not just various cases of crooked teeth.

For the visual exploration, we'll leave the treatment coordinator's office and get the patient to a dental chair, where we'll hand him or her a mirror and explain what we're looking for, as well as address questions such as:

- Is the patient dentally ready?

  ▫ That is, if he or she is a child, are there enough teeth, or if an adult, are all the teeth present and healthy and ready to receive orthodontic appliances?

  ▫ If we are dealing with an adult, are there any other dental issues that need to be addressed *before* any orthodontics can be done?

- Is there a dental or functional need?

  ▫ In other words, is there a condition that, if left unaddressed, can become a problem now or later?

- Is there an aesthetic need or desire for treatment?

  ▫ Has the patient or parent expressed concern about a visual issue, such as too much spacing or teeth sticking out?

If the answer is "yes" to one or more of these questions, then we'll likely make a recommendation to pursue orthodontics.

If we do recommend treatment, the next step is to bring the patient into the treatment coordinator's office and summarize once again what we found and what we recommend going forward. If it's braces, the treatment coordinator will typically spend some time showing the patient how braces go on and how an expander goes on if one is necessary. If we're recommending Invisalign, we'll also review how that product works and how we use the company's proprietary software, ClinCheck, to show you a 3-D rendering of how your teeth would move using this system.[2]

Then, because we believe in the power of the visual and tactile, we also have models of teeth with braces, with Invisalign, with retainers, and without anything on them—all so that patients can familiarize themselves with their treatment and, in doing so, demystify the process. We spend whatever length of time the patient needs to understand what we're recommending and why.

Lastly, we also have a bank of images of thousands of patients we have treated over the years. While each one is a unique and special individual, chances are that we have treated someone with a similar malocclusion and can bring up pictures of the patient's bite before and after treatment. We have found that patients really appreciate being shown similar cases to theirs, as it helps them visualize the outcomes they can expect. It also gives them a reference of how long they should expect to be in treatment.

---

2   In chapter 9 we'll talk about the iTero system, which is an exciting new way to make digital 3-D images of patients' mouths. This can be used to gauge tooth movement over time—*and* to create retainers and Invisalign trays, if needed.

MAKING SURE WE ALL HAVE THE
INFORMATION WE NEED

We always allot enough time in our initial consultation appointment to take a full set of orthodontic records, including extra-oral and intra-oral photographs, intra-oral scans, digital models of your teeth, and panoramic and cephalometric x-rays.

Each patient walks out with a folder full of information about the practice, the doctors, a financial plan explaining insurance coverage and out of pocket expenses, and a detailed plan as to what to expect from his or her orthodontic treatment.

When you begin treatment with us, you get what we like to call our "to-go" or "goodie" bag. This bag is modified constantly and contains anything from a toothbrush and floss for the adults, to a toothbrush and a toy for the kids as a "thank-you." We know our patients have made a sacrifice in their schedule to be with us, and we like to express to them how much we appreciate the time they've given us.

In the ideal world, that first office visit should take somewhere between half an hour and forty-five minutes. We know our patients are busy, and sometimes just finding the time to come in and see us can be a challenge. It is for this reason that we have scheduled our new patients' visits in a way that they can oftentimes get their braces on or even be scanned for Invisalign that same day. However, there is never any pressure to start; we do this purely out of convenience and consider it another way in which we can offer a higher level of service and a value-added option to our process. No matter what, we make sure the patient is comfortable before we do anything.

KEEPING THE DENTIST IN THE LOOP

One important piece of information we ask every patient to share with us is the name of his or her regular dentist. This serves two purposes: one, it allows us to send a "thank you" letter to him or her for referring that patient to us, and two, it lets the dentist know that this patient is now undergoing orthodontic treatment.

Once we open that line of communication, we can begin to address specific concerns with each other. For instance, if I notice an impacted tooth on a mutual patient, I'll let the dentist know to keep an eye out for it during the patient's next visit. Or if the dentist has information about the patient's long-term growth patterns, he or she may let us know to better inform the orthodontic treatment. On any given day we may see several patients who are not quite ready for orthodontics. A seven-year-old, for instance, may greatly benefit from removing some baby teeth while waiting for orthodontic treatment, so the pediatric dentist would get the okay from us in the form of a written or digital letter to do so. We'd refer the patient back to have these teeth out, and the patient would be served well by the open dialogue between her two dental providers.

At a minimum, we have three points of contact with the regular dentist for each of our orthodontic patients:

1. Right after the first consultation

2. When we put braces on

3. Right before we take braces off[3]

---

3   This final check-in, right before the braces come off, is to get the dentist's input in case there's something special about that case and, at the very least, give him or her the heads-up that the patient will need a post-orthodontic checkup and cleaning.

A fourth and final point of contact is done in writing, when we send the dentist a letter letting him or her know that the patient's appliances have been removed.

> Open communication keeps orthodontist and dentist in the loop, so that we can ultimately provide that patient with the best comprehensive treatment possible.

This open communication keeps orthodontist and dentist in the loop, so that we can ultimately provide that patient with the best comprehensive treatment possible. At the heart of it, the patient wins.

THE BEST AND THE BRIGHTEST

Concerning our staff, we do everything we can to attract and retain the best and the brightest. This goes for the doctors we work with as well as the clinical and support staff, including our orthodontic assistants, front-desk people, and treatment coordinators. To do this, we emphasize the importance of continuing education in three key ways:

1. Because of the volume of people we see, our facilities are great places to learn. In most businesses, the best places to learn are at the best and busiest because you're taught through experience.

2. We assure that all our people have the proper certification before they start with us and that they maintain that certification over the course of their employment.

3. A requisite of employment with us is that our employees participate in continuing education. This could include sending our treatment coordinators to a conference on

how they can work better with the OrthoFi system or sending our doctors and clinical assistants to educational opportunities such as the Greater New York Dental Meeting to attend courses. We also bring lecturers in to speak to our staff and conduct internal training on the latest techniques; whatever we can do to promote continuing education, because every pearl of knowledge that someone gains adds to the value of our services and what we can offer our patients.

When you give people the skills to treat your patients better, then your outcomes improve—from the individual-patient level up to the impact-on-the-whole macro-level. Patients have a better experience, staff is better trained, and everyone is more confident. When staff members perform better, they're paid more, and eventually they use that training to move up or laterally or to a different practice. They develop a valuable skill set that they can take with them. We get feedback all the time from our staff on how important that is and how much they appreciate it.

The Importance of Work Ethic

While we're constantly looking for the best and the brightest staff members, we aren't necessarily looking for those who are gifted in dentistry when they start. Sometimes the best people are those who are simply willing to work, so we look first at an individual's work ethic and his or her ability to comply with and conform to our in-office culture. Maybe a candidate doesn't have ten years of orthodontic experience under his or her belt but *does* have a bright personality and a fierce hunger to learn. We've found that candidates with these qualities are more likely to do far better at their job than seasoned veterans who are set in their ways.

Our hiring practices are as much of a personality evaluation than a clinical one. We believe that the people who want to, can. If you want to learn how to be the best assistant in putting on braces, you can. If you love engaging patients and parents, we put you in a position where you can do that.

Before we began hiring based on personality and desire to learn, the challenge we so often ran into was a disconnect between what we read in someone's resume and what they were like in person. Now we explain to candidates that our offices are a family atmosphere. We may be a little dysfunctional sometimes (as every family surely can be at times), but our goal is quality care and growth of the individual employee. Our staff members work with and for each other, which means that after someone is "hired," it's the current staff that either confirms that hiring process—or does the firing. Our staff, we've found, are willing to work with good, like-minded people who treat our patients the right way. Good people bring out the best in everyone, so when we hire someone new, we hope that person can stand with our goals and vision, which is to be polite, to deliver quality care, to work well with colleagues and the doctors.

Here are a couple of our core values that emphasize the importance of work ethic:

Enthusiasm—Happy and enthusiastic staff have a profound effect on patient experience and that, in turn, translates into making patients partners in their treatment and enthusiastic ambassadors for our practice and brand.

> **Opportunity**—We believe in giving our wonderful employees the chance for upward mobility and growth within our organization through investment in their education and profession development.
>
> *See the "Our Services" page for all our core values.*

Our offices hire slowly and fire quickly, and if there's an ability for good staff members to grow outside of our offices, then we're happy to help them do better and set them free. It's a wonderful thing when former staff can talk about your organization with others and tell them how much they learned with us and how much they grew as individuals. Those are our ambassadors, because there's no better recommendation than one that comes from someone who has nothing to gain from it—they're just happy with their experience and want others to enjoy the same. You can't fake that kind of excitement.

We want anyone who gets on the phone with us to know that, even if it's a little crazy at our offices that day, the person they're speaking with loves his or her job. So, we focus on finding, training, and retaining the kind of people who love what they do and are hungry to learn more. We want those people to be our first points of contact with our patients—because you never get a second chance at first impressions.

We also want our patients to know that, in a day and age when we're all so busy and things need to be done yesterday, that we're doing our best to be available at times that work for them. If that means delaying an appointment while you're studying for exams or traveling to another country, we can do that. We're also open early, late, and on weekends to accommodate as many different schedules as we can.

On any given day, our offices are a busy, buzzing atmosphere, but it's the calmly controlled, efficient kind of atmosphere that only places with happy, well-educated staff can pull off!

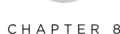

CHAPTER 8

Retention for Life

By Seth Newman, DDS

Regina gave me an abashed grin when I asked her what brought her into the office.

"I'm here because I didn't listen to my orthodontist twenty years ago, and now I'm paying for it," she said. "I didn't notice it for the longest time, but over the past year it's felt like my teeth have started to, I don't know, kind of slip out of proper alignment and are slowly crashing toward one another, you know? And then suddenly I distinctly remembered being a freshman in college and tossing my retainer as far as I could throw it in celebration of my new freedom and getting out from under 'The Man.' But now I'm certainly regretting that decision."

I smiled. "Well, if it helps, you certainly aren't alone," I said. "More than half of the adult patients we see had braces when they were kids, and by and large, their experiences were the same: they had braces, they wore their retainers for a while, and eventually they gave up on wearing them at all or just slowly forgot about them. Then things started shifting around in their mouths and that's why they're back in our office in their thirties, forties, or fifties—to treat the shift that occurred because they stopped wearing their retainers."

Everything changes as we age, I explained, so it's not unreasonable to think that your teeth will change and move with time, too. In fact, it is an absolute given that our teeth will move over time, which is why we believe in our "retention-for-life" protocol—a program that includes the redundancy of both cemented lingual retainers and removable clear retainers.

The challenge we run into, however, is that patients who come in because their teeth have shifted over time believe that all they need are new retainers and they'll be set to go. But that's just not the case. Retainers, by definition, retain teeth in a static position; they don't have the ability to move them.

"Ah," Regina sighed. "Then I can't just get a new retainer and be on my way, can I?"

"Not if we're going to get your teeth back to being healthy and straight," I replied. "But the good news is that since you did have braces earlier, we likely won't need to do a full, comprehensive treatment; maybe just some time in Invisalign or some limited orthodontics for a few months. But let's look and find out."

Regina's misunderstanding is a common one. Retainers are so tied in our minds to braces that many of us naturally assume that they also move our teeth. That is, if we forget to wear them for a while (or for years), we often think we can just snap them back on and they'll push our teeth back into their ideal bite. But retainers just aren't built to do that.

Regina was fortunate. Her teeth only experienced minor movement that put them about 15 percent off of what would be an ideal bite for her, so we were able to put her in a spring aligner—which looks like a retainer but with a spring wire that presses against the back of the teeth to bring them into alignment—and then in a retainer, which she promised to wear much more diligently.

However, it is important to know that her case is the exception to the rule. In fact, she was very lucky.

When patients come in with minor movement such as Regina's—say, 10 or 15 percent off what would be ideal for their oral and facial structures and smile—and are not interested in fixing the discrepancy, oftentimes we'll make them a new removable retainer that will keep their teeth from veering any more off center.

As orthodontists, we believe that everyone should have perfectly straight beautiful teeth, which is why we usually recommend bringing them back to ideal, either with something as simple as a spring aligner or, if it is more involved, braces or Invisalign. Once everything is back to looking amazing we will more than likely recommend that they have a fixed retainer put in so that they never have to worry about it again.

DO I REALLY NEED TO WEAR MY RETAINER?

Using braces to move teeth is a dynamic process. When you first got your braces off, it probably felt like a huge relief—like taking off a cast or as if someone suddenly stopped squeezing you in a gigantic hug. All those pressures were gone. But because your teeth were gradually moving for a year or more, they were not entirely set in place when those braces came off. They need to be held firmly in place for the greater part of the first year after braces (or the removal of any other appliance) to give the bone time to solidify around the roots of the teeth in these new positions. And if your teeth were particularly crowded or crooked, or took longer to move into an ideal position, the more likely your teeth are to relapse to some degree if simply left to their own devices.

This is where the retainer comes in, as its sole purpose is to hold the teeth in place until they're firmly set, and then to keep them there.

As Regina found out, the body is constantly changing, and teeth shift right along with it. If you go for too long without a retainer, chances are that you'll have to go through a re-treatment with an aligner or even spend some time in braces to correct your bite before you can be fitted for a retainer again.

Believe it or not, we take as much pride in your new smile as you do. You are our billboard! So, when someone's teeth shift out of an ideal position that we all worked hard to create, it can be disappointing. Forget that it is a blow to our egos—redoing something that you already did, and that took a while to do, can be frustrating, and no one enjoys the "re-treatment" conversation.

For this reason, we are huge advocates of retention, and we stress this importance with our patients when their braces come off. Our standard retention protocol is to have a lower permanent retainer placed in addition to clear, removable aligner retainers. Where possible, we also try to place the permanent retainer on the lingual surface of the upper front four to six teeth. After a short time, we ask that our patients only wear their removable retainers at night. We find that this is enough time to ensure that your teeth look as good as when you first completed your orthodontics. It also eliminates the risk associated with retainers, the main one being that they can be lost or accidentally thrown out with a meal. This happens more than you would think with patients who wear their retainers during the day. At the very least, having a permanent retainer placed on the lingual surface of the upper and lower front teeth gives you insurance in the form of time that you can use to get back to us for another impression and a new retainer.

The clear aligner retainers, also called Essix, look like an Invisalign aligner and are made of hard, durable plastic so that they can't distort. There's no wire over the teeth, either, so they're highly esthetic and very comfortable. We find our patients really love them, especially since they do not have the look or feel of a traditional retainer. These retainers typically last anywhere from two to five years, with some patients being harder on their retainers than others. For instance, some patients grind their teeth at night while others may play with them by snapping them on and off. On the other hand, some patients may keep their retainers immaculate and end up getting a significantly longer life out of them.

Here is a little secret that most orthodontists don't tell you: While we can take an educated guess based on where a patient started, we really don't know for sure whose teeth are going to relapse and whose will stay perfectly aligned. There are patients who experience relapse, and I am surprised by how much their teeth shift, while others have very little movement based on where they were when they started.

We recommend wearing a retainer for not one or two years, but for the rest of your life after braces. And that's where the value of fixed retainers comes in.

Therefore, we recommend wearing a retainer for not one or two years, but for the rest of your life after braces. And that's where the value of fixed retainers comes in.

Take the story of Roxana, who came in one day to have her wisdom teeth checked and to make sure her permanent lower retainer was still in good working order. I knew that she had completed her orthodontics a little more than three years prior, and I was impressed by how great her upper teeth looked. However, when I complimented her on this and on how well she was doing with her retainer, she looked me right in the eye and said, "Doc, I haven't worn that thing in years."

That kind of retainer lapse is a gamble, and it looked like lady luck was on her side. While many of our patients are Roxanas and don't follow the recommended instructions, we are always going to advocate that our patients wear their retainers.

WHAT IS A FIXED RETAINER AND HOW DOES IT WORK?

It's likely you've seen plenty of people with fixed retainers and not even known it. In fact, the people wearing them have likely forgotten that they even have them. This is because a fixed retainer is really nothing more than a small metal bar bonded to the back of the teeth. It's comfortable and there are no extra pieces, such as wires, that can break or degrade over time.

When we tell our patients about these permanent retainers, the question we usually get is, "So this retainer is going to be on me for the rest of my life?" The honest answer is that the longer you have it on, the better. Permanent retainers are so named because only an orthodontist should remove them. We love permanent retainers, because they are not subject to our moods and memory. They are glued in around the time that braces are removed and are placed behind the lower (and sometimes upper, as well) front teeth. The lower front teeth have the shortest, smallest roots, which means that they're more likely to shift over time due to their smaller foundations. If we look at someone who had previous orthodontics and was not the most diligent about wearing retainers, without a doubt, it's the lower front teeth that have started to shift.

Simplicity and permanence are the two biggest reasons we recommend a permanent retainer. With a traditional retainer, there's not only the risk of losing it, but also the risk of the retainer distorting or breaking over time. The patient may not even notice it for a while, during which time the teeth may begin to shift. We have also found that as patients wear their retainers more and more sporadically, they do not notice the subtle changes that happen and can generally get the retainer to "fit" —until they cannot. By that point, unfortunately, it's already too late, as the teeth have shifted beyond a point where they are readily correctible with a retainer.

The one downside to a permanent retainer is that it can make flossing more challenging, which is the main reason some patients don't like them. While you can floss around them, you do need to be more diligent with the practice, and you may need the aid of a floss threader. On the plus side, the consumer-dental-products market has responded to the prevalence of permanent retainers. There are products such as super floss, which is designed to be stiff enough to aid in threading floss between the teeth, and special flossers that use a jet of air and water to remove plaque. In the end, however, we believe that traditional floss is still the gold standard.

Fixed or permanent retainers are usually only placed on the lower front teeth, not the upper, for two reasons:

1. A permanent retainer is limited to the front teeth, so it does not do as good a job of holding a widened smile as a removable retainer would.

2. The biting force of the lower teeth on the upper teeth tends to lead to more upper-retainer breakage.

As convenient as they are, it is our feeling that permanent retainers are not a total substitute for the removable versions, as they can only be placed on the front teeth and don't do anything to retain the side or back teeth. In addition, often when we're straightening someone's smile we're also widening it, and without something to hold the new smile in place, the potential for teeth to shift is significant. For this reason, we typically ask a patient to wear a removable retainer along with the permanent one, as it's the combination of the two—the full retention of the removable and the long-term insurance of the permanent—that will keep teeth looking amazing for years to come. When our patients are compliant with these instructions, we see almost no shifting, even years after we're done.

We do have some patients who elect not to have a permanent retainer, though we usually discourage this. Typically, patients choose to go without a permanent retainer for the freedom of it. Even though the permanent retainer becomes virtually unnoticeable over time, some people still prefer the freedom of being able to take the retainer out entirely whenever they choose.

Who Doesn't Need a Fixed Retainer?

With our youngest patients—the ones undergoing Phase One treatment—we normally don't recommend permanent retainers, as their canines and other side teeth are still erupting, and some movement of the teeth around them is needed. We usually give these patients removable clear aligner retainers or classic Hawley retainers, the kind most people picture when they think of traditional retainers. Once our young patients lose their baby teeth and their adult teeth start growing in, we usually tell them to stop wearing their retainers so that all their adult teeth can properly grow in without interference. Once they have their full adult dentition, we can determine if they need a new retainer or require any additional orthodontic treatment.

WHAT IS THE RETENTION-FOR-LIFE PROGRAM?

While the first few years after braces are the most critical, when you're prescribed a retainer, it's a lifetime commitment. It's a lot of work on the part of both the patient and the doctors to get those teeth straight and into an ideal bite, so to help preserve that work, we began our Retention-for-Life program.

Apart from the normal wear and tear that our most popular retainers—the clear aligners—undergo every day, life also happens. Retainers get lost, stepped on, chewed on by dogs, and thrown in the toilet; you name it, we've heard it! The most memorable instance for me was when a patient's grandmother thought it would be a good idea to boil his retainer to get it clean.

Another one of my more memorable stories was when a patient, Richard, lost his in the course of becoming an adult:

He got braces for the first time in college because, in his words, "My parents never got around to it." He wore upper and lower clear braces for thirteen months, always following instructions and never breaking a bracket. As a result, he finished his treatment five months earlier than anticipated. However, even though he was a model patient, he elected not to get a permanent retainer.

"I love to floss too much," he told me. "You don't have to worry about me."

He really believed this and so did I, but two years later, Richard came in to see us because his teeth had shifted. He'd lost his retainer two moves ago and in the excitement of graduating from college and entering the job market, he didn't get a replacement. He was embarrassed, but also not looking forward to wearing braces again because of his lapse in retainer wear. Fortunately, while he did need re-treatment, it was only for his front teeth, which we were able to straighten out in only ten weeks. And this time, he happily went with the permanent retainer!

It's frustrating to have to pay for replacement retainers, and we never feel good about having to charge patients for something they paid for already. That's why, when we heard about this program that our colleague, Dr. Jamie Reynolds, was using, we jumped on it.

"Retention-for-Life" is basically an insurance policy for your retainer. Patients simply pay a one-time fee and nominal co-pay any time they need new retainers for the rest of their lives. With this system, any time they need a retainer, they can come in and have one made. Some patients come in once a year, some come back every five years. There's really no limit on how often they can get their retainer replaced, which we've found helps quite a lot when it comes to the worry of potentially breaking or losing a retainer. If one goes missing or is chewed or otherwise destroyed, our patients are much less likely to hesitate about coming in for a replacement; this means less time out of a retainer and much less risk of teeth shifting too much before the replacement is made.

While we can't say that all our patients are as diligent with their retainers as we would like, we have had quite a few who are. One patient, Geovane, got his braces off when he was thirteen years old. His was a tough case, and we worked hard to give him an ideal smile. He wasn't the biggest fan of his braces, but even though he was young, he appreciated how hard we worked to give him an amazing smile.

When his braces came off, we had the same discussion we have with all our patients regarding the importance of wearing his retainer. Happily, Geovane got the message and was still wearing his retainer regularly at age twenty-two, which was the last time he came in for a retainer replacement. It was his third set, the first one wearing out by age sixteen and the second one breaking when he decided to use it as a mouth guard while lifting weights. This latest one had been lost in a move, but since he was part of the Retention-for-Life program, he had no worries about getting a replacement quickly and at minimal cost.

CHAPTER 9

Straight to the Future: Technology and Orthodontics

By Efstathios Giannoutsos, DDS

The world, as I write this in 2018, is a completely different place than it was in 2008, and it will be completely different again in 2028—which is why staying on top of technology is a core value to our practice. Every minute of your time is precious, and the more efficient we can make one of your visits, the more value you'll get out of the time you spend with us.

There was a time in the not-too-distant past when a visit to the orthodontist took at least an hour and a half out of your day, and that usually didn't include travel time. Having to spend that kind of time on anything, especially when you have to do it every three to four weeks, just isn't fun—but it doesn't happen nearly as much anymore. Instead, we're working on ways to reduce the time of your visit to thirty minutes, max, where practical. In fact, it is not uncommon for some patients to have fifteen-minute visits for a quick examination of their braces or Invisalign. That would be the total time in the office from check-in to check-out.

We can do this by streamlining the process as much as possible, while also creating a balance so that your visit doesn't feel rushed and you leave with a full understanding of what was done and what to expect at your next visit. If we've done our job right, the only steps you have to take when you arrive at our office are those first few through the door and into the treatment room.

DIGITAL APPOINTMENT BOOKING

Most of our patients are tech-savvy, or at least have some familiarity with smartphones and online services, and the way we interact with them is constantly evolving. Whereas one patient may prefer to book an appointment in person or with another human being over the phone, more of our clientele prefer a completely automated booking process. Whether you prefer to e-mail us, text us, or even chat with us online, we've got you covered.

The ability to make an appointment with us is as easy as clicking on "contact us" or "make an appointment" on our website. The form that appears lets you choose from your best time of day and best days of the week, then provides you with options on available times. And remember, if it's a first visit, that initial consultation is completely free.

The next step is where the technology gets even more impressive. This is where we get rid of the clipboard and move you from a state of fifteen minutes of paperwork to an entirely paperless welcome to our office.

THE NO-CLIPBOARD WELCOME ROOM

The exchange of information is a given at any first-time visit to a doctor's office, and it's not something that patients look forward to. The process of filling out form after form can be a time drain, especially if the first time you're seeing all that paperwork is when you walk in for your appointment.

Rather than spending forty-five minutes having people run around with your insurance card, making copies of it, getting on the phone, and talking to the insurance company, we use the OrthoFi system, which allows new patients to provide us with all their necessary information securely and in the convenience of their homes or offices.

This allows us to take care of the administrative portion of your first visit before you even arrive for their appointment. Plus, it gives the clinical staff time to review your medical history and insurance information so that once you arrive, we can get straight to the business of addressing orthodontic needs.

On the day you come in, we have everything ready and we can get right to the business of understanding what they need from both a treatment and cost perspective. (Don't sweat it, however, if you aren't able to fill out the forms ahead of time! We understand that life can get in the way, and for that reason we have plenty of iPads in the office, so you can take care of it then.)

This may seem like a nice option and a good time-saver to the average patient, but to the clinical staff, this is a revolutionary advancement. What most patients don't know is that we once had to budget at least thirty minutes per patient to process their information when they arrived. With the information already filled out and confirmed, that time has gone from thirty minutes to zero, and the only thing we need to worry about once you walk in is getting to know you and making sure you have a wonderful experience in our office.

CUSTOMIZED COMMUNICATION

Another practical feature of our increasingly digital communication system is that patients have the option to tailor their methods of contact to whatever serves them best. If you prefer all email, we can do that. If text is better, that's perfectly fine. We can even do both if you're worried about missing a reminder. Of course, we still have staffers who will happily answer the phone during office hours if you prefer booking appointments in person, but you don't have to. And that also helps eliminate the time spent waiting for someone behind the front desk to get off the phone when you're at the office.

Which leads to our next piece of streamlining tech—the check-in kiosk.

FROM SLIDING WINDOW TO SWIPING RIGHT: DIGITAL CHECK-INS

So much of the check-in and check-out processes at the orthodontist office is simple routine. From confirming your information to booking your next visit, there are multiple steps that can be handled just as easily—and more quickly—when you can take care of it yourself.

Take the tedious task of transferring information from clipboard to computer. If forms aren't filled out online, a front-desk person is tasked with transferring the information from handwriting to digital records, which takes time both for the transcriber and for the patient, who must wait until his or her medical records are updated and confirmed before seeing the doctor. Instead, by having a self-check-in option at a kiosk, patients can confirm their arrival and verify any updates to their medical information with a few clicks.

Online forms, digital kiosk check-ins, and medical information verifications aren't just timesavers for the front desk and patient; they also give the doctor an opportunity to prepare for the patient in advance, so that instead of being updated about a nickel allergy after the patient has been sitting in the treatment room for five minutes, for instance, the doctor knows about it beforehand and already has suggestions on alternative options. And since the forms include an update on your insurance information, the clinical staff can also give you a total understanding of how any changes to your benefits will affect the treatment's cost, and what that means for your payment plan.

Our goal is to get to the point where patients don't necessarily need to speak to the front-desk person at all, if they don't want to. Instead, patients can go to the kiosk after seeing the doctor and, if the recommendation is to come back in four weeks, for instance, this data is already in the system. Then when you log in, you're immediately given options for available appointment slots at that time. You can just pick the day and time you want and confirm it. We have also recently implemented chair-side checkout and booking of your next appointment, with an instantaneous email or text confirmation so that you are set to go even before you go!

Payment, too, is done automatically through the online OrthoFi system, unless otherwise specified, so you don't have to stop and pay on your way out. Again, these may seem like small steps, but when you add them up they equal significant time savings for both the patient and the office staff. Just like in any business, the more automated we can become, the less manpower we need for tasks such as sending out statements and collecting payments. This translates into more efficiencies for us, and more savings that we can pass along to our patients.

FROM STICKY GOOP TO SCANNERS: 3-D TEETH AND JAW MODELING

On a more technical level, along with being able to store and update patients' digital records, including x-rays and images, we're also able to create models of the teeth and jaws more efficiently using advanced 3-D scanners. Patients no longer have to endure that awful, sticky, artificially flavored goop that they once had to bite down on for minutes at a time to make a mold of their teeth. Now we use an advanced iTero scanner to create a highly accurate 3-D scan of the teeth, which can be used to gauge tooth movement over time and to create retainers and Invisalign trays, if needed. Additionally, these scans can be used to 3-D print any of the previous states of your teeth with perfect accuracy and precision. It's a perfect, permanent electronic record of your condition—and, if at any point we need to refer back to the state of your teeth at any earlier point in treatment, we have it ready to go.

What's also remarkable about the scanner, apart from eliminating the inconvenience of old-fashioned dental impressions, is that it allows both the doctor and patient to see a 3-D rendering of the bite in real time as it's scanned. Compared to the set time it used to take per arch with dental impressions, the scanner is a huge time saver.

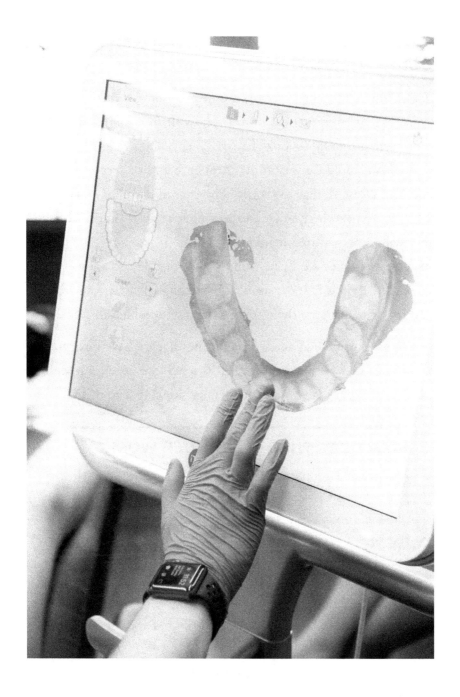

CAN YOU SHOW ME HOW MY TEETH ARE GOING TO LOOK? YES, WE CAN!

This is one of the most remarkable aspects of this technology. For years, our patients have asked us to show them a simulation of how their teeth are going to look after treatment. Until recently, however, the best we could do was to dig through banks of previous patients and find a case similar to theirs. Now we can accurately show them a projection of where we can expect their teeth to finish, and how that will look, within a matter of minutes. It's akin to the way that new-buyer homes are being built, where people can virtually walk through their new home instead of just sitting down with an architect and trying to visualize their house from a set of blueprints.

We are so excited about this feature that we have incorporated it into our new patient experience. Patients love getting to see how their teeth are going to look and we love showing it to them.

HOW DOES THE 3-D SCANNER WORK?

The scanning process is remarkably simple. We ask the patient to sit as still as possible in the dental chair as we glide a specialized scanning wand over the surfaces of the oral structures and teeth. The images taken by the wand are sent directly to a large screen, which displays the scanning process in real time. As we've grown accustomed to the device, we've been able to get our time down to about two and a half minutes for a complete, accurate scan.

This was a huge benefit to one of our patients, Cynthia, who couldn't stand the old method of bite impressions and plaster modeling. Cynthia really wanted to be fitted with Invisalign, but a bad experience with a dental

impression, where some of the thick alginate accidentally went down her throat, leaving her with a bad taste
in her mouth in more ways than one. Then one day, when
she came in with her daughter, Geniane, she saw us use
the scanner and was shocked.

"You can do impressions without the goop?" she asked.
"Wow, that's pretty amazing."

A few days later, she came in to be scanned for Invisalign,
and she's been a raving fan of the technique ever since.

HIGH-TECH ORTHODONTIC MATERIALS

Apart from the scanner, we also make it a point to use appliances that
are at the pinnacle of technological advancement. Whether it's the
latest in hypoallergenic and biocompatible adhesives and brackets,
or the thinnest, yet strongest iteration of nickel titanium wires for
braces, by staying on top of the latest innovations, we're able to
give our patients options that are less bulky and more effective than
their dated counterparts. Ultimately, this helps us move teeth more
quickly and cut down on the number of visits that patients need to
make before their treatment is complete.

There are so many other technological advances at our disposal
as of this writing that were merely a wish only one generation earlier.
We have coated wires, for instance, that almost perfectly match the
color of the teeth, and mono-crystalline sapphire clear brackets that
draw out the color of the underlying tooth to make the braces almost
perfectly invisible.

Then there are the "passive" braces systems, such as Damon. By
"passive," we mean that instead of using small rubber bands around

each bracket to hold the wire in place, the brackets are outfitted with a small sliding door that does the job. This eliminates the tension and friction caused by the rubber band, and significantly reduces the chair time needed for the patient. Some systems use both passive and active braces, such as the In-Ovation system, which works some inherent elasticity into the brace itself so that the clinician can optimize the movement of the forces on the teeth.

PARTNERS INSTEAD OF PATIENTS

Even though most patients don't really care to get into the esoteric minutia of our practice, digitization allows each of them to be much more involved and in control of the orthodontic process. This transparency, as well as a greater degree of interaction and revolutionary time-saving techniques, makes the entire process run much more smoothly and allows us to view our patients less like "patients" and more like partners in a therapeutic alliance.

Time is exceedingly precious in the rapidly increasing pace of our world, so every minute we can shave off of someone's visit becomes valuable. We want the time that you spend with us to be efficient and productive. We don't want you to feel as though you had to rush through paperwork but rather that you actually had the time to talk with your doctor and clinical staff about your concerns. To do this, we continue to look toward the future to make each minute you spend with us today is even more valuable.

CORE VALUES

Partnering and becoming active members in the communities we serve, providing opportunities for professional growth of our team and enhancing our patients lives and smiles are essential to our missions as dentists. Here are our core values we live every day in our practice:

Respect—Providing an environment where our team treats patients and one another with respect, kindness and dignity.

Diversity—Recognizing the beauty in the vastness of our differences. Fostering a culture that celebrates what makes us unique and embraces and recognizes this as an opportunity to learn from one another.

Sustainability—Taking the lead in assuring that the materials and methods we use are kind to our environment and limits our footprint.

Growth—Understanding that fulfilling our mission and maintaining a clear path to continually honoring our core values requires fiscal strength and profitability.

Appreciation—We love our patients. We sincerely appreciate the trust they have placed in us and are grateful every day that they have given us the opportunity to practice a profession we love with an amazing team made up of wonderful individuals.